MENOPAUSE

MY EXPERIENCE IS MY STRENGTH

BHAGIYALAKSHMI MUKUNDAN

Clever Fox®
PUBLISHING

Chennai • Bangalore

CLEVER FOX PUBLISHING
Chennai, India

Published by CLEVER FOX PUBLISHING 2025

ISBN: 978-93-6707-911-9

INDEX

PREFACE

Do you recall lying awake at 3 a.m. inside a labyrinth called menopause and wondering how in the world you arrived there, struggling with so many physical and emotional trials? I do. It was 2003, and I was adrift in the tumultuous waters of this life transition, overwhelmed by the sudden appearance of symptoms for which I had no explanation.

It was a journey of discovery and healing, driven by the need to find solace and a solution. I did many hours of research, numerous conversations with medical professionals, and a rigorous commitment to self-care. In all this, I discovered a pathway that brought me to a new sense of well-being and empowerment.

This book is a testimony of my personal experience and a lighthouse of hope to women who are still lost in the maze called menopause. I wish someone had given me this wonderful guide, rich with practical suggestions, personal experiences, and valuable insight when I began my journey.

I believe every woman deserves to feel confident, capable, and empowered regarding her health and well-being.

I want to help and empower other women who are experiencing a hard time with menopause. Sharing my journey and some practical takeaways, pieces of advice, I wish to provide you with a roadmap for a healthier, happier, and more rewarding life for women in need.

Remember, you are not alone. We can face the challenges of menopause together, with grace, resilience, and a renewed sense of purpose.

CHAPTER 1

UNDERSTANDING MENOPAUSE

It was more of a rude jolt to the system, my menopausal awakening. One morning, I woke up all disoriented and very fatigued. Just making a cup of tea seemed like the biggest task in front of me. And in such times of agony, when I was struggling with my changing body, I realized that after all, I was not alone. Millions of women worldwide were suffering from similar symptoms.

The medical fraternity often isolates menopause as a purely biological phenomenon, largely confining its definition to hormonal alterations. But in reality, things are much more complicated. Menopause represents a change that touches every sphere of a woman's life: her physical and mental health, as well as her emotional well-being.

Finding My Way

Determined to have my health and happiness back, I set out on a searching journey for knowledge and support. I went through extensive literature that existed concerning menopause. I consulted gynecologists, psychiatrists, and all those who could offer insight and advice.

My research opened my eyes to how holistic the approach towards managing menopause really needs to be. I learnt about the connectedness between the mind, body, and spirit, and how one has to nourish each of these three factors to help the body work at optimum capacity. Besides, I discovered just how powerful self-care can be and how crucial a supportive environment is.

My menopause has been a life-changing experience. It has taught me the roles of resilience, self-compassion, and personal empowerment.

What is Menopause?

Menopause: a word that's frequently spoken and met with wrinkled brows. Let's make that adjustment. Menopause, like puberty or pregnancy, is simply a natural stage of a woman's life cycle. Your body is trying to tell you to relax since it has gone enough.

Think of menopause as the final chapter in a fantastic book. This is the phase where the main character finally has time to think things through, unwind, and relish the rewards of her life's adventure. It is an opportunity for growth above all else, but it is also about change.

Symptoms of Menopause

Many of them are annoying, and it seems that menopause has its share of tricks. Night sweats and hot flushes are two of the most typical concerns.

Imagine you're enjoying a quiet, calm moment when suddenly, you feel like you've been dropped into a sauna. That's a hot flash. The nighttime equivalent is night sweats, which can wake you up completely drenched. It's like your body decided to take an unannounced steam bath.

Mood Swings: Happy, Sad, Hungry, Guilty?

Hormonal fluctuations can take one's emotions on a rollercoaster ride. At one moment, you might be laughing, and at another, crying. It's like having a drama queen living full-time inside a person. Don't worry; you are not alone. Much like you, the majority of women experience mood swings when they approach menopause.

Sleep Disturbances: Catching Zzz's Can Be Tough

Sometimes, during menopause, sleep seems to be far away. This is often due to either night sweats or flashes, or because the mind is constantly on overdrive. It is as if your body has forgotten how to switch off at night.

Vaginal Dryness:

Vaginal dryness is a very typical menopause symptom. It is a source of major discomfort for women. But then again, don't worry about it; we are going to discuss that a little later on in more detail.

Physical Changes: Your Body is Changing

When you reach the menopausal stage of your life, your body changes. You may very likely start to experience some changes in your skin, hair, and weight. It's just as though your body is reshaping itself.

Though these are common symptoms, it does not mean that it's like that for everyone. Some other symptoms of menopause in women include joint aches, headaches, and difficulties in passing urine.

Remember that these symptoms can vary in severity and duration, too. Some women will sail through menopause without a hitch and hardly any symptoms, but some will face much more significant issues. The important thing is to listen to your body and seek support if needed.

The Stages of Menopause

First, let's split it into stages to understand the period of menopause more clearly.

- Perimenopause: That is just the opening act. Your ovaries get into a slower pace in the production of estrogen, and you may start to feel a little different. Irregular periods, mood swings, and the occasional hot flash might start making an appearance.
- Menopause: This is the big event. You've reached menopause when you've gone 12 consecutive months without a period. It's the official end of your menstrual cycle.
- Postmenopause: This is the final act. You are past menopause, and while some symptoms might still linger, you are officially in a new chapter of your life.

Hormonal Changes: The Culprits and the Heroes

Those little chemical messengers, hormones, play a big role in menopause. Estrogen and progesterone are the main players. As your ovaries wind down, their levels start to drop. And that may cause a little ripple effect throughout your body.

Don't worry, though. While these hormonal changes can bring some challenges, they also open doors to new possibilities. More on that in the sections to follow.

There you go – an overview of Menopause. Its part of life, and the time has come to talk about it openly and honestly. Let us, together, break the myths attached to this phase.

Hormones are truly the unsung heroes—or villains, depending on the day—of our bodies. They are just tiny chemical messengers zipping around inside us and having a say in everything that our bodies can do. And when they start partying—as they seem to do in menopause—things tend to go a little nuts.

Estrogen: The Queen Bee

The hormone that rules females is called oestrogen. It affects everything, including bone health and the menstrual cycle. Your ovaries start to produce less oestrogen as you get closer to menopause. The main source of many of the difficulties associated with menopause is this slowness.

Your Body in Flux

Think of your body like a house. Now, estrogen acts as the 'cement' that holds it together. When estrogen levels fall, it's like yanking out some bricks. Let's look at how this affects various rooms in the house:

- Skin: Estrogen keeps your skin plump and supple. Lower levels of estrogen mean your skin might get drier, less elastic, and wrinkle-prone. Just imagine the paint fading off your house's outer surface.

- Bones: estrogen contributes to the health of bones. Bones deteriorate and osteoporosis risk rises as it falls. Imagine that the foundation of your home begins to deteriorate.
- Heart: Estrogen is thought to protect your heart in some way, though this is not completely known. Your risk of heart disease may rise if your body produces less estrogen.
- Brain: Concentration, memory, and mood are all influenced by estrogen. Mood swings, forgetfulness, and loss of focus can all be caused by fluctuations. It resembles an electrical short circuit in your house.
- Vagina: The lining tissues of the vagina and the urinary tract are maintained in excellent health by estrogen. Women who have low levels may experience dryness, irritation, or even difficulty urinating. Of course, every woman's experience is very different. For some, it seems to sail through changes with hardly any upheaval, while others are challenged by more significant difficulties.

Awareness of how these hormones change can help us navigate menopause with some understanding and grace. In the next section, we'll cover the emotional part of menopause.

The Emotional Rollercoaster

The challenge of menopause encompasses not just the alterations you are experiencing in your physical body. It's a phase of ups and downs, emotional upheavals. Picture your emotions like riding a rollercoaster, moving with exhilarating highs, terrifying lows, and unexpected twists and turns.

Mood Swings: Emotional Maelstrom

Hormonal swings might give you the impression that your feelings are travelling at breakneck speed—you might be laughing one moment and sobbing the next. It's as though your body is naturally endowed with a drama queen. Although mood fluctuations might be perplexing and upsetting, keep in mind that you're not alone. This phase of the menopausal process has been completed by many women.

Anxiety and Stress: Feeling Overwhelmed

During menopause, anxiety and stress can feel overwhelming. This is often a result of physical symptoms like hot flashes and disrupted sleep. You may find yourself constantly worrying about your health, appearance, and future—as if your mind is running a marathon without any preparation.

Depression: The Silent Struggler

While moodiness is a common feeling, continuous feelings of being down, hopeless, or worthless may indicate that one is depressed. You can easily get this mixed up with normal ups and downs of mood swings, which makes clinical depression seem shallow. If you need any help, reach out to a healthcare professional.

Grieving and Identity

This makes it a clear demarcation for many women of the close of their childbearing years. There may be a sense of loss, with accompanying grief, due to this sense of finality. Your sense of self could be so identified with being a mother or partner that it is difficult to negotiate these changes.

Building Resilience

Remember, you are not alone in your feelings. So many women go through this. It involves building resilience by coping with stress in a healthy manner, having self-care techniques, and getting support from friends, family, or a therapist.

This is a time of transition, so it is quite normal to feel mixed and overwhelming emotions at menopause. When you know what's going on and how to get support, you'll sail through this phase of your life with elegance and strength.

Mitochondria: The Powerhouses Within

You will wonder, "What do tiny cellular powerhouses have to do with menopause?" A lot, it turns out. Dubbed the "powerhouses of the cell", mitochondria play a role that is very critical in energy production and overall health of the cell; its functioning goes deep into the intricacies of menopause.

Understanding Mitochondria

Imagine your body as a bustling city. Mitochondria are like the power plants that crank out juice for every action that goes into life—from contracting muscles to firing brain cells. These tiny structures inside your cells convert your nutrients into adenosine triphosphate, or ATP—the energy currency of the body. The Mitochondria-Menopause Connection

Research points increasingly toward a mitochondrial function associated with menopause. A decline in estrogen level seems to have some impact on the health of mitochondria, which then causes a chain reaction effect of signs and symptoms of menopause. Here is how mitochondrial dysfunction explains the symptoms of menopause, from energy depletion to others:

Energy Depletion: Lowered mitochondrial activity can cause energy depletion, which most women experience during menopause. You will not be so energized if your cells' power plants are not running full tilt.

Metabolic Changes: Mitochondria are in the process of turning food into energy for the body. In case mitochondrial function is not up to the mark, weight gain may occur at the very least, which will further create metabolic disturbances common in menopause.

Oxidative Stress: The mitochondria are the major site of formation of reactive oxygen species, which can induce cytotoxic effects when there is an imbalance. Estrogen is among the most important molecules, due to its antioxidant properties, that can quench Reactive Oxygen Species. Hence, their reduced levels increase oxidative stress further, increasing the multifactorial risk associated with aging and various diseases.

Cellular Aging: Mitochondria play a key role in the aging process. A decline in their efficiency can accelerate aging, which may manifest in various ways, such as skin changes, loss of muscle mass, and cognitive decline.

Bone Health: Mitochondrial function goes a long way in maintaining bone health. However, estrogen deficiency alone could promote the loss of bone mass with osteoporosis if associated with mitochondrial dysfunction.

Mitochondrial Health Improvement

Although mechanisms are yet to be precisely elucidated, here are steps for mitochondrial health during menopause.

- Diet: Focus on good food intake, like all those rich in antioxidants. Try adding foods that may be of more direct benefit to the functioning of the mitochondria, such as fatty fish, nuts, and seeds.
- Exercise: Any regular exercise will have a more positive effect on mitochondrial function. Just combine some aerobic cardiovascular exercises with resistance training.
- Stress Management: Long-term stress is a killer to mitochondrial health. Practice some forms of relaxation, be it meditation or yoga, and deep breathing exercises that help in reducing stress.
- Supplements: Some supplements, primarily CoQ10, alpha-lipoic acid, and acetyl-L-carnitine, are being studied for their potential benefits on mitochondrial functions. Consult with a healthcare professional before initiating new supplements.
- Sleep: Repair and regeneration of mitochondria are necessary, and it's crucial to have sufficient sleep. Aim for 7-9 hours of sound sleep each night.

Yes, the relationship between mitochondria and menopause is still relatively under-explored. Isn't it exciting to know enough about it to take control of an important life stage and start building toward better well-being?

Embracing the Journey of Menopause

Involving hormonal, physical, and emotional changes in a very intricate way, menopause is just an ordinary part of life. Hormonal, physical, and emotional changes go side by side in a very complex way. It is hard, yet it is a time to mature, discover the self, and develop resilience.

Knowing the physiology behind menopause, particularly in the realm of hormones and mitochondrial function, is helpful for treating the symptoms that accompany this transition. From hot flashes to mood swings, bone health, and energy levels, these physical changes may drastically affect a woman's quality of life.

One has to approach menopause from both a physical and an emotional perspective. Looking after your body through good diet, exercise, and stress management can help to support the health of mitochondria and reduce some of the physical challenges at this life stage. Equally important is the need to tend to your emotional landscape through seeking support and building resilience.

Remember, menopause is a journey, not a destination. It's about finding a new definition of self, celebrating your strengths, and finding new passions. Equipped with better knowledge of the phase, more self-care, and positive vibes, you can stridently pace through this stage of life with confidence and class.

Let us embrace menopause as a total natural transition that it is, and empower women to engage in this new phase with vitality and purpose.

Easy-to-Remember Tips: Chapter 1 – Understanding Menopause

1. **Learn the Basics** – Understand menopause is a natural phase.
2. **Know the Signs** – Look for changes like hot flashes and irregular periods.
3. **Track Changes** – Keep a diary of symptoms for better awareness.
4. **Stay Informed** – Read or consult professionals about hormonal changes.
5. **Expect Variability** – Recognize that menopause affects everyone differently.
6. **Embrace Change** – View menopause as a new chapter of life, not an end.

CHAPTER 2

STRESS: MENOPAUSE'S UNWANTED ROOMMATE

Once I had almost reached my late 40s, excessive stress was what finally got the better of me, with the onset of menopause. It was as though physical and emotional changes were just attacking me at once: sleepless nights, mood swings, and anxiety became constant companions. I felt like I was losing control, with everything starting to take its toll on my work and personal life.

I knew I had to get back on track and find my peace. After months of searching and reflecting, I came across the Inner Engineering program by Isha Foundation, founded and run by Indian yogi, Sadhguru. There was something in the techniques and practices taught in the program that made sense to me, particularly the fact that breath work is the most significant method for controlling the body's stress response.

By making the breath work a regular part of my routine since that program, it helped to bring my stress levels down gradually, and I improved my sleep patterns. The once-looming anxiety became much more manageable. Day by day, I was feeling more balanced, mentally and physically.

I would highly recommend Inner Engineering for every woman going through menopause. Breath work and control of the vagus nerve have changed my life, as I am sure they can be yours, reducing all that stress and health havoc going on with this stage of life that menopause can raise.

Stress—there goes the unwanted visitor, who seems particularly fond of making themselves at home during menopause. Perhaps it sent itself an invitation that we never sent out, you would suppose. Let's examine the relationship between stress and menopause and explore some solutions.

Stress might sometimes make menopause symptoms worse. And the never-ending cycle makes one feel overwhelmed.

Menopause symptoms, including mood swings, hot flashes, and nocturnal sweats, can be made worse by stress. It can exacerbate the situation by introducing sleep interruptions into the mix. Your body releases the hormone cortisol while under stress, which can cause sleep disturbances and increase the dreaded hot flashes.

How Stress Impacts Your Body

Although the psychological effects of stress are highly popularized, equally prominent are its damaging effects on physical health. Chronic stress acts like a silent disruptor, slowly and systemically weakening the immune system, therefore making it much more susceptible to a myriad of illnesses. In doing so, it continues to heighten the risk of creating major health problems, such as heart disease and hypertension. Moreover, it also does not spare the digestive system. Stress can cause Irritable Bowel Syndrome and increase the severity of other gastrointestinal disorders.

Skin health, too, declines under constant stress. The body's reaction can manifest in the form of breakouts, rashes, or even eczema. Not only this, but stress also increases the rate at which a person ages by developing premature wrinkles and other symptoms of early skin aging. Further, it is sleep-disruptive; insomnia adds yet another health problem to the list. It is hence very important to identify these physical signs of stress to deal with them before things go out of hand, ensuring overall health.

Managing Stress During Menopause

So what can you do to manage your stress during menopause? Here are some effective ways to do so:

- Mindfulness and Meditation: These activities might help in calming your mind and reducing stress. A few minutes of deep breathing exercise will work wonders.
- Physical Activity: Exercise is an efficient and strong stress-buster. Do what you like—dancing, swimming, or hiking.
- Healthy Eating: Feed your body good food to balance your mood and energy levels.
- Good Sleep: Get plenty of restful sleep. Engage in a calming pre-bedtime routine to help relax your mind and body.
- Time Management: Stress can result from feeling overwhelmed. Break tasks into smaller steps.
- Social Support: Spend time with supportive friends and family. It is surprising how helpful just talking about your feelings can be.
- Professional Help: If stress is really having a tight hold on your life, consider talking to a therapist or counselor. Keep in mind that asking for help, reaching for support, is a key step in starting your healing journey.

There is no one right way to respond to this; it is all part of the stress management process. As a result, try out several tactics to see which ones perform best for you. You will experience an improvement in your mental state as well as your physical and general well-being if you take action to lessen stress.

Stress Reduction: Your Path to Calm

Stress is a constant companion for so many women, and menopause can put that shadow under klieg lights. Let's explore tools to banish this unwanted guest.

Yoga brings together dynamics of physical movement with breath work and meditation into a complete strategy for the alleviation of stress. The poses recommended for the nervous system are forward folds and the child's pose. From dancing to swimming, exercise releases endorphins—the mood-boosting chemical.

Meditation is training the mind in concentration. The most powerful methods are through guided meditation, mindfulness, and body scans. Positive thinking can be cultivated through gratitude journaling and visualization. Power relaxation, tensing, and releasing the muscles really helps ease the tension in the body.

Get enough sleep with a routine, sleep-conducive bedroom, and no screen time before lights out. Basically, what works is a routine. Small changes, like a daily walk or minutes of meditation, can have a big effect.

Your mind and body are one; take care of both to help prepare for the optimum condition for sailing through menopause.

The Power of Yoga

Apart from physical postures, yoga is a whole practice where both body and mind meet. Physical activity, breathing practices, and meditation are all joined together in a way that allows one to be relaxed and at peace with oneself.

- Physical Benefits: The relaxation in muscle tension, increase in flexibility, and enhancement of the energy level in the body go without saying. In this way, regular practice of yoga is bound to ease typical menopausal symptoms of joint pains and fatigue.
- Mental Benefits: Practicing yoga sharpens focus and concentration on the present moment while releasing oneself from bothersome worry. The asanas can reduce feelings of anxiety, thus elevating mood and the general feeling of well-being.
- Specific Poses: Some yoga poses are particularly beneficial in the cause of stress relief. Forward folds, child's pose, and bridge pose supported by a block help to calm down the nervous system.

The Joy of Exercise

It can also decrease stress, improve sleep quality, enhance energy levels, and even alleviate symptoms of anxiety and depression, especially after regular exercise, since exercise releases endorphins, which are natural elevators of the human body.

- Find Your Groove: Find activities that you enjoy; this could be dancing, swimming, walking, or biking.
- It's all about the intensity: Aim for a mix of cardio and strength training.
- It's All About Consistency: Even bursts of exercise throughout the day make a difference.

Meditation: Stillness and Serenity

It will help you train your mind, focus on your thoughts, and concentrate. It is living in the present moment—the 'now'. By meditating regularly, one will notice a decrease in the level of stress, an improvement in concentration, and an improvement in emotional well-being.

- Guided Meditation: Guided meditations may be of use to beginners. There are tons of applications and resources available online.
- Mindfulness meditation: Focus on breath and sensations without judgment. Such a simple exercise could turn out to be powerful.

- Body scan meditation involves noticing different parts of your body and releasing tension as you go.
- Tapping into the Power of Positive Thoughts
- Your thoughts have so much to do with how you're feeling and your general well-being. Learning positive thinking techniques can make all the difference.
- Challenge Negative Thoughts: If some negative thoughts come to your mind, question the truth behind them and then let positive affirmations flow in.
- Gratitude Journaling: It focuses you on what you are grateful for, changes your angle of view, and may lighten your mood.
- Visualization: See yourself relaxed and free from stress. This may help drive away your anxiety and help you feel more relaxed.

Power Relaxation: Your Body's Reset Button

It is the process of tensing and relaxing different muscle groups to release physical tension. The technique can be performed either in a seated or lying-down position.

- Progressive Relaxation: This technique involves focusing on tensing and releasing various muscle groups, beginning from the soles up to the head.

- Quick Relaxation: In case one has no time to practice it fully, he should learn to tense and release his hands, arms, and shoulders.

Aligning Your Body Clock

A disturbed pattern of sleep can exacerbate the stress and symptoms of menopause. Prioritize quality sleep with:

- Establish a routine: Go to bed and get up at the same time each day, even on weekends
- Make a sleep-supportive environment: Keep your bedroom dark, quiet, and cool
- Turn off electronics: The blue light in handheld electronics has been implicated in interfering with sleep.
- Management of Caffeine and Alcohol: Do not consume in excessive amounts in the late part of the waking day.

Remember, you are on the journey of change in your life through incorporating these mechanisms in reducing stress and not the destination itself; accordingly, have compassion for yourself and take time to notice when you have moved even in the small steps of change. Put differently, by concentrating on self-care and decreasing stress, you are opting to live a better life.

Your Body's Internal Clock: The Importance of Circadian Rhythm and Sleep

Imagine all of it to be like an orchestra. Every organ—with your heart and mind as its major players—comes together to generate harmony: that's what your body is. And leading the symphony is your circadian rhythm—an internal clock governing propriety and decency, telling you when to sleep, wake, and carry out other functions of the body.

This 24-hour rhythm is mainly driven by light, but factors such as diet, exercise, and stress can also function as significant influences. Your circadian rhythm, in combination, controls when you are ready to pay attention and be active and when you are prepared to be sleepy. Disruption, though, leads to a cascade of negative outcomes.

Sleep is a time for your body to repair, grow, and rejuvenate. From consolidating memories to boosting immunity, good health relies on sleep to carry out its functions. Hormonal changes during menopause easily disrupt sleeping patterns because of hot flashes, night sweats, and a change in the circadian rhythm.

A dysregulation in the circadian rhythm can cause a truckload of problems, from weight gain and mood swings to weakened immunity and cognitive difficulties.

Therefore, prioritizing sleep and life structuring in harmony with one's natural circadian rhythm can really improve the quality of one's life, both during menopause and thereafter.

The Maestro Within: Your Circadian Rhythm

It's like the internal clock of your body, which normally runs independently according to its self-dictated circadian rhythm—a self-sustaining, oscillatory process for periods of approximately 24-hour activities in the body. Not only does it control sleep/wake cycles, but it also controls hormone secretion, body temperature, and even digestion. Light, however, is a major factor in dictating this rhythm. Diet, exercise, and social contacts do have a bearing on it as well.

If your circadian rhythm is aligned, you have boundless energy, are focused, and well rested. But when it gets knocked off, everything that can go wrong does.

Sleep: The Body's Restoration

Sleep is foundational to a proper circadian rhythm. It is during sleep that your body tends to restore tissues, build muscle mass, and consolidate memories. This also forms the time when important hormones such as growth hormone and melatonin are secreted.

In this way, menopause often disrupts sleep through hot flashes, sweating at night, and hormonal changes. This will start to misalign your circadian rhythm again, spiralling into a vicious cycle.

Staying in Step with Your Circadian Rhythm

If you want to be as healthy as possible and to feel the best you can during menopause, respect your body's need for natural rhythms. Here are some tips:

- Establish a regular sleep pattern: Every day, even on weekends, go to bed and wake up at the same time to set your body clock.
- Make a sleep-friendly environment: Dark, cool, and quiet are the bed compartments. Buy comfortable bedding and develop a relaxing routine before sleeping.
- Keep control over light exposure: Expose yourself to light in the morning to set your circadian rhythm. Avoid excess use of screens before sleeping because it interferes with sleep due to its blue light.
- Regular Exercise: Physical activity is known to enhance sleep quality. However, avoid high-intensity exercises immediately before sleeping.
- Watch What You Eat: Avoid heavy meals before bed, and drinks that have a lot of caffeine. There are

some foods that naturally contain melatonin, like cherries, and such foods will make you drowsy.

- Take Few Naps: While long naps are refreshing, they ruin night sleeping.
- Manage Stress: Stress interferes with our ability to rest. Add relaxation techniques like meditation or yoga to your daily routine.

The Impact of Disrupted Circadian Rhythm

Because of this, a desynchronized circadian rhythm can be behind several kinds of issues. Some of them could be;

- Mood Disorders: Anxiety and depression are caused due to loss of sleep and circadian rhythms.
- Metabolic Problems: When sleep is irregular, the hormone balance in the body will be affected due to desynchronization, leading to an increase in weight and finally, to metabolic issues.
- Weaker Immune System: Your immune system depends on sleep. If you sleep poorly over a long period, your body might become prone to infections.
- Poor Cognitive Functioning: Sleep deprivation causes poor memory capacity, concentration, and indecisiveness in individuals.

Incorporating sleep and the body clock does much to ameliorate the overall well-being during menopause.

Conclusion

Your body is such an amazing tool that, of course, like any well-designed system, it works best under ideal circumstances. No one can overstate the importance of paying attention to and trying to respect your body's circadian rhythm during the phase of menopause. Improve all aspects of your life significantly by putting sleep at the top of your priority list: creating a suitable environment for sleeping and tailoring your lifestyle to your natural circadian rhythms.

Remember that little changes can have great effects. Setting up a regular sleep practice or relaxing with leisurely thoughts before going to bed imparts how one can regain her sleep and thus really improve her living quality.

As we pass through menopause, self-care becomes ever more important, and for the first time, we may really listen to our bodies. With a good understanding of the intricate connections between sleep, circadian rhythm, and overall health, you are making a conscious move toward an enjoyable and healthy life.

Easy-to-Remember Tips: Chapter 2 – Stress Management and Menopause

1. **Breathe Deeply** – Practice daily relaxation techniques.
2. **Exercise Regularly** – Use physical activity to reduce stress.
3. **Set Boundaries** – Avoid overloading yourself with commitments.
4. **Sleep Well** – Prioritize restful sleep to manage mood swings.
5. **Try Mindfulness** – Meditate or use yoga for mental clarity.
6. **Talk It Out** – Share stressors with friends or professionals.
7. **Limit Caffeine and Sugar** – Avoid substances that elevate anxiety.

CHAPTER 3

HOW CAN NUTRITION AFFECT YOU?

Going through menopause, I was soon to learn it wasn't only the hot flashes, mood swings, and sleepless nights that I had to handle, but that my diet was equally as important. Menopause is the period of drastic change within one's body, whereby most of what we eat influences the way we feel.

The relationship between diet and menopausal symptoms is not something one would really be involved with or consider in the past. Like many of us, I had assuredly presupposed that as long as I was eating reasonably well, I really had nothing to worry about. But as the symptoms of menopause began to take hold, I began to see just how vital balanced nutrition is.

The Role of Diet in Combined Menopausal Symptom Management

Let's face facts: Menopause sucks. Your hormones are on a rollercoaster, and your body is trying to reset to a new "normal." It is like you are going through puberty all over again, except this time around, you have a mortgage to pay and probably a couple of kids to take care of as well. It's not the most fun time, honestly.

What finally clicked with me was how much my diet was affecting my symptoms. An itch, irritation, tiredness, and hot flashes came in the wake of selected foods, while, otherwise, with healthier alternatives, I felt better. In essence, my body was trying to tell me something, and I finally decided to listen.

Some of us may sail through menopause, but most of us have one thing in common: how our bodies react to food. Our metabolism slows down after menopause; hence, we experience increased body weight—especially around the torso. Our body also becomes more sensitive to the change in blood sugar levels, which may increase cravings and mood swings. And then, of course, there is the consideration of our bones: menopause can cause bones to thin, so calcium and vitamin D become even more vital.

This is where nutrition comes in. By focusing on a balanced diet, you can help your body and manage your symptoms as your body transitions. Think of this as giving your body the right tools to see it through all these changes.

Importance of Balanced Nutrition (Aligning with "BNI")

When I say the words 'balanced nutrition', it is not just a buzzword. A balanced diet is a type of diet where your body will get the level and type of nutrition it requires to perform functions flawlessly. Well, it's very much like a car because it needs a proper mix of fuel, oil, and coolant, meaning everything is in perfect working balance.

In my opinion, the BNI is more of a guiding principle. It's not about calorie counting or not having a plate of pasta. It's about understanding what is actually in the food you are putting in your body. It is about having the right mixture of proteins, fats, carbohydrates, vitamins, and minerals.

A balanced diet is important during menopause for the following reasons:

- Hormonal Balance: One should consume such nutrients that help maintain hormone balance, and hormone levels would be at a crisis level during menopause. For instance, fat, particularly healthy fat found in foods like avocado, nuts, and seeds, is an important raw material that is useful in the production of hormones.

- Bone Health: It is also very important, as bone density gets diminished when estrogen levels fall. Sufficient intake of calcium and vitamin D should be ensured. One can keep one's bones healthy by consuming leafy greens, almonds, or fortified dairy products.
- Mood Stability: The fact might just be beyond belief, but food can actually have a direct impact on one's mood. It's been documented that, generally, the intake of foods rich in Omega 3 fatty acids—salmon and seeds, among them—may even help reduce depression or anxiety throughout menopause.
- Energy Levels: The hormonal imbalance due to menopause often leaves one feeling tired, and it is at these times that sufficient nutrition can give your flagging energy levels a kick. Complex carbohydrates in the form of whole grains and legumes provide a steady supply of energy without the crash associated with refined sugars.

This will condition your body with the right nutrients and help it respond to the stress and rhetoric from menopause in a far better manner. It's all about making your body resilient, and it begins with what you put on your plate.

Develop Insulin Sensitivity and its Advantages

One issue related to menopause that was important upon reading was insulin sensitivity. Insulin is a hormone within your body that you utilise to regulate the amount of sugar levels in your blood. Your system may become a little more insensitive to insulin during menopause, which raises the amount of sugar in your blood, which in time will pose a high risk of developing type 2 diabetes.

While I was trying to manage myself, I came across a program conducted by Dr. Tripathi. This was called 'Freedom from Diabetes Program'. I was enrolled in this program for one year, which helped me manage my insulin sensitivity, without any medication.

But the good news is, one can become insulin sensitive only by diet and changes in one's way of life. For me, this was empowering, for it meant I could take charge of my health rather than be at the mercy of my bodily changes.

- Eliminate Refined Carbohydrates: Food such as white bread, sugary cereals, and pastries tend to increase the sugar levels in the blood without any considerable latency. This, in turn, develops insulin resistance. I replaced them with whole grains like quinoa, brown rice, and oats.

- Increase Fiber Intake: Fiber slows the rate at which sugar enters the bloodstream, evening out those peaks of blood sugar. I made sure to include plenty of fruits, vegetables, and legumes in my diet.
- Healthy Fats: As I have said before, healthy fats are great at producing hormones, but on the other hand, they tend to make one insulin-sensitive. I started incorporating more omega-3 fatty acid sources in my diet, which included things like fatty fish, chia seeds, and walnuts.
- Stay Active: Other things that may help increase insulin sensitivity include exercise. I find that adding regular physical activity to my day, whether it is just a brisk walk or a session of yoga, makes all the difference in how I feel.

In turn, being focused on these areas, I felt that there was more energy in my body and that I started to feel better. Normalized blood sugar made me feel in control, and instead of fighting my body, I was working with it. The building of insulin sensitivity has helped to work with menopause symptoms and reduce the risk of long-term health issues.

Focus on Whole Foods and Mindful Eating

As I ate my way through menopause, I learned that it wasn't just what I ate but how I ate it. This is where the whole food and eating concept collided with each other. This approach, or shall I say, "Focus on Ur Food U Cat," is a playful way to remind one to pay attention to what and how you eat.

Whole foods are nothing but those foods in or closer to their natural state: fresh fruits, vegetables, whole grains, nuts, seeds, and lean proteins. Nutrient-dense foods can be replete with nutrients, fiber, and healthy fats, hence promoting the management of menopausal symptoms.

Eating mindfully is the process of being present while one eats: relishing every bit of food, paying attention to hunger and fullness, and not distracting oneself with TV or a smartphone during the meal-just a few ideas.

I started with this practice of mindful eating, whereby I felt so in tune with my body and its needs. I enjoyed it more and found that I overeat less and make unhealthy choices less often.

Here's how I found a way to fit those whole foods and mindful eating into my life.

- Eat the Rainbow: A rainbow of fruits and vegetables began to fill my plate. Since each colour represents different nutrients, I knew that by eating a variety, I had a good mix of vitamins and minerals.

- Read Labels: Anytime I had to buy food that came in a package, I intentionally read food labels. I picked out foods with short and pronounceable ingredient lists and bypassed things with added sugar, artificial flavours, and preservatives.
- Practice Gratitude: I thanked God for the food in front of me before each meal. That little practice was one that helped me to slow down and appreciate my meals more.
- Listening to my Body: I took cues from my body in terms of hunger and fullness to eat when I'm hungry and stop when I am satisfied and not consume food because I have always done so at this time of the day.

By focusing on whole foods and learning to eat more mindfully, I found that I had more energy, fewer cravings, and a better feeling of well-being. It wasn't about adherence to a strict diet; it was about making choices that nourished my body and mind.

Personal Dietary Changes and Their Impact

These dietary changes were no mean feat, but the quality of life that ensued had to be taken into account. I remember well one of those days when the pressure of menopause took on an entirely new meaning. I was totally beset with a craving for comfort food that was completely off the charts in terms of how overwhelming it was. Though it could have been so easy, in those moments, to reach for something fried or sugary, just to emotionally self-soothe with food, that time I did otherwise—I put my new habit into practice.

Instead, I whipped up a healthy meal of whole grains, lean protein, and a ton of veggies. I cooked it slowly before sitting down to eat, and really enjoyed my food. To my surprise, not only did the meal hit the spot for my hunger, but it also elevated my mood. I felt calmer, centered, and prepared for the rest of my day.

That was the moment for me. It was a reminder of something that I have known very well: food is not only a power source but actually a medication. The right foods can balance our hormones, stabilise our mood, and support our overall health through menopause.

A ripple effect began to echo in all other aspects of my life. I found that I can more readily maintain an active lifestyle. The mood was leveled, and that alone brought much power to all of the other areas in my life, especially with regard to relationships with family and friends. Even my sleep improved, something that I have struggled with since my youth.

Of course, the pathway was not smooth. Somewhere along the way, I would slip back to old habits or make less healthy choices. But I didn't beat myself up about it. Instead, I framed every meal as a fresh opportunity to feed my body well and to make a good choice.

Ultimately, the changes I made to my diet had a significant impact on my menopause journey—helping me manage my symptoms, improve my health, and feel more in control of my body. And the best part? These changes weren't about deprivation or strict rules. They were about adding more of the good stuff-more nutrients, more mindfulness, and more joy.

But now, as I look back at this part of my life, it actually was a journey of another discovery. I learned to listen more attentively to my body, what it needed, and how to feed it with proper food. Through that, I found a sense of balance again.

So, if you are amidst menopause and it is becoming unbearable, I encourage you to take another look at your diet. All it takes are little things that make a big difference. Eat nutritionally; develop your insulin sensitivity; pay attention to whole foods; and become a mindful eater. It is not about perfection; it is about finding what will work for you and then doing the best you can through making choices to support your health and happiness. I'm telling you, your body will thank you.

Easy-to-Remember Tips: Chapter 3 – How Nutrition Affects You

1. **Balance Your Plate** – Include proteins, healthy fats, and complex carbs.
2. **Boost Calcium and Vitamin D** – Protect your bones.
3. **Hydrate Often** – Drink plenty of water throughout the day.
4. **Eat Mindfully** – Avoid overeating and choose whole foods.
5. **Avoid Processed Foods** – Cut down on sugar and refined carbs.
6. **Include Antioxidants** – Add berries, greens, and nuts to fight inflammation.
7. **Check Iron Levels** – Replace what your body needs during menopause.

CHAPTER 4

LIFESTYLE FACTORS AND MENOPAUSE

The changes I faced in menopause weren't really about just what I ate but rather how I lived my everyday life in total. And though I have always loved the concept of a balanced life, menopause taught me just how important some of the lifestyle factors could be in making certain symptoms bearable and one's life reasonably manageable. In this chapter, I have discussed some of the major lifestyle changes that really helped boost my energy levels: exposure to sunlight, grounding techniques, physical activity, and energy healing.

The Significance of Sunlight Exposure

We all know that we feel happier when we have spent time in the sun, but during menopause, it becomes even more important to do that. During my journey through ups and downs, I gradually realised just how important this incorporation of sunlight into my daily rhythm was.

The Importance of Sunlight for Bone Health

Vitamin D is essential for calcium absorption in the body and is crucial for maintaining bone strength. Alongside an absence or low level of Vitamin D, the amount of absorbed calcium decreases in the body, therefore increasing the risk for bone-related problems.

Research proves this liaison. In fact, in an article in 'The Journal of Clinical Endocrinology & Metabolism', it was concluded that postmenopausal women with higher levels of Vitamin D have higher bone density compared with those with lower levels. Another article in *Osteoporosis International* sheds light on the well-known fact that vitamin D deficiency is highly prevalent in menopausal women, and that appropriate sun exposure is crucial for preventing bone loss

Sunlight and Its Effects on Mood and Energy

But its benefits aren't confined to just your bones. I realised that besides the good changes in my physical health, my mood and energy level also significantly improved from exposure to the outdoors and sunlight. Sunlight initiates the release of serotonin, a neurotransmitter associated with mood regulation, sleep, and appetite. Higher levels of serotonin relate to feelings of well-being and happiness, which may be particularly beneficial during this time since mood swings are a common accompaniment of menopause.

And scientific evidence proves this effect, too. One study published in *The Lancet* said that the more natural light there is available, the better the mood of a person will be, which means symptoms of depression decrease. This comes in handy during menopause since fluctuations in hormones may alter mood regulation. Days out in the sun, spent outdoors, made me feel more positive and resilient, even at the mercy of the emotional roller coaster part of menopause.

Balancing Sun Exposure for Optimal Benefits

Of course, with everything in life, it's all about finding a balance. While sunlight is great, too much of it does cause skin damage and increases one's risk for skin cancer. These risks weighed against each other; I had always tried to be out in the sun either early in the morning or late in the afternoon when the UV rays weren't strong. That way, I could enjoy the sunlight without its negative side effects.

The American Academy of Dermatology advises seeking shade and wearing protective clothes during the peak sun hours between 10 a.m. and 4 p.m., besides using sunscreen that is SPF 30 or higher. By following these recommendations, I was able to enjoy the sun's benefits without being worried about damage to my skin.

A Positive View of Sunlight During Menopause

Being able to incorporate sunlight into one's life can help greatly with realising such health benefits throughout the menopausal life stage. In fact, from good bone health to much-improved mood and energy levels, sunlight is relatively free and easily accessible. By learning how to understand these benefits from a scientific perspective and practising sun safety, it can be guaranteed that sunlight will become a large part of your menopausal life, as it has in mine.

Techniques of Grounding or Earthing

Another lifestyle factor that took me by surprise for how it affected my menopause journey was grounding, also called earthing. It does sound a little "out there," but bear with me—grounding is a very uncomplicated practice with some pretty powerful benefits.

This involves direct contact with the Earth through walking on grass, sand, or soil with bare feet or an invention of mats and sheets to cover your bed with the view of imitating the Earth's natural electric charge. It was thought that by coupling with the Earth's energy, we can balance our body's electrical systems and, thereby, reduce inflammation, improve sleep, and even enhance mood.

I was sceptical the very first time I heard about grounding. After reading up more on the potential benefits and how it could help with stress, anxiety, and sleep, which were issues I faced at a point in my life-I decided I would give this technique a try.

First, I started by taking a few minutes each day to walk outside barefoot in the garden. The first week or so felt weird, almost childish, but after a while, I did begin to notice some of the more subtle changes. I slept better: falling asleep faster, waking up more rested. I felt my levels of stress decrease. I simply felt that I was more in touch with the world around me, more present, and less hounded by all these concerns that had been eating at me.

The science is still emerging, but the idea is that the Earth's surface has a negative electric charge and when we are in direct contact with it, we allow those electrons to flow into our bodies, neutralising free radicals and reducing inflammation. Now, whether scientifically proven or not, what I do know is that grounding made me feel better. It became a meditative process for me- a time to stop, breathe, and commune with nature. And those few moments were worth their weight in gold during the crazy days of menopause.

Oil Pulling

Oil pulling is a traditional Ayurvedic method that has gained popularity due to its simplicity and effectiveness in promoting overall well-being. It is especially beneficial after menopause, when hormonal changes occur and toxins accumulate in the body.

Swish a spoonful of natural oil—typically coconut, sesame, or sunflower oil—around in your mouth for 15-20 minutes. It is said to "pull" toxins from the body via saliva, thus improving dental health and overall detoxification.

Oil pulling provides numerous benefits to menopausal women. It promotes gum and tooth health, which might be influenced by hormonal changes. It can help reduce inflammation, strengthen the immune system, and aid digestion—issues that are frequently present during this period.

The best time to perform oil pulling is first thing in the morning, on an empty stomach, before brushing your teeth. After swishing, spit out the oil (never swallow it, as it contains the toxins removed) and rinse thoroughly with warm water.

Including this easy habit into your daily schedule is a subtle but potent approach to support the natural detox processes that the body undertakes during menopause, and further support well-being.

Dry brushing

Dry brushing is a simple yet effective activity that promotes lymphatic drainage and overall health, particularly during menopause. Using a natural bristle brush, softly stroke your skin upwards, beginning at your feet and working your way up to your heart. This approach stimulates the lymphatic system, aiding in cleansing, lowering fluid retention, and potentially increasing blood circulation. It also exfoliates dead skin cells, leaving your skin smooth and refreshed. For optimal results, add dry brushing to your morning regimen before taking a shower. Combining this with hydration and a healthy lifestyle will maximise its advantages and help your body's natural cleansing processes during this transitional period.

Positive intentions while drinking water

Infusing happy intentions into drinking water is a simple but transforming technique, particularly during menopause. Before drinking a sip, pause and think about an encouraging statement or affirmation, like "I am strong," "My body heals," or "I embrace balance." This thoughtful behaviour can help you connect more deeply with yourself and your body's needs. Water, the essence of life, serves as a conduit for fostering happiness and mental well-being. Combining this habit with proper hydration throughout the day will help your body's natural functioning and improve mental clarity. Small, focused steps like this can have a significant impact on this journey to healing..

Physical Activity and Its Benefits

If there is one thing that I learned through menopause, it is that physical activity is a 'cherry on the cake'. I know, I know; the last thing you want to hear is the need to exercise when all you want to get through are those periods of hot flashes, fatigue, and mood swings. But trust me, being able to maintain yourself as active makes quite a difference.

During menopause, our bodies are subject to great change, where we lose muscle mass, our metabolisms go down, and we gain weight much more easily around the belly area. Regular exercise can counterbalance such changes and even enhance metabolism, preserve muscle mass, and help control body weight.

However, the benefits of exercise are not only physical. In my experience, exercising helped prevent the buildup of stress and irritation. A short walk or a yoga session often made a difference when I felt grumpy or anxious.

Exercise releases endorphins—the body's natural 'feel-good' chemicals—which help manage the emotional highs and lows that are so common during menopause..

A combination of exercise types worked best for me. Here's how I broke it down:

- Cardio: The most common activities that work your heart continuously, such as walking, swimming, or cycling, were excellent for keeping my heart rate up and calorie burn steady. I always tried to get the recommended amount of at least 150 minutes a week of moderate-intensity cardio for overall health.
- Resistance Training: We all lose muscle naturally with age; that can slow our metabolism and cause increased accumulation of fat. To combat this, I made sure to include strength training in my routine by lifting weights, using resistance bands, or carrying out bodyweight exercises twice every week.
- Flexibility and Balance: Yoga was the way I incorporated into my journey to good flexibility and balance, aspects that decrease as one gets older. It also offered me relaxation from my busy mental life and a way to centre myself.
- HIIT Workouts: I have also tried HIIT workouts, consisting of very short bursts of high-intensity exercise followed by rest or low-intensity periods.

Such workouts are great for cardiovascular fitness in a relatively short length of time.

I only tried to do more of what I enjoyed and was able to stick with. I didn't do exercises that I hated because if it wasn't fun, I knew I wasn't going to keep up with it. Instead, what I did was try to find movement that felt great for my body and my mind. The result? I felt stronger, more energised, and more in control of my body, even though menopause was bringing about its changes.

Yoga

Menopause is generally viewed as a natural but no less challenging period in women's lives. In that respect, yoga and energy healing can make such a transition much easier, more balanced, and even empowering with their holistic approach.

Yoga, mainly focused on mindfulness, breathing, and soft movements, is one of the best options to lighten many menopausal symptoms. Regular practice can help alleviate most complaints, such as hot flashes, mood swings, and sleep disturbances. For example, forward bends, inversions, and supported postures cool the body, quiet the nervous system, and promote relaxation. Visualise being in a quiet room, stretching softly, when all of a sudden, it feels like stress melts away- what a calming exercise it is.

And that, my friend, is the magic of yoga: how it manages to balance all the energy systems within our bodies, especially in times of hormonal roller coasters. Yoga stimulates the parasympathetic nervous system, which is responsible for sending messages to our body that we need to relax and reduce stress. And stress plays an enormous role in worsening the symptoms of menopause! This means you will not only feel more relaxed but also better prepared for those unpredictable mood swings or that one surprise hot flash that always seems to strike at the most inopportune moments.

Here are 2 asanas that can help relieve menopausal symptoms. While these are being described here for your understanding, you are strongly advised to practice these asanas under the guidance of a Yoga instructor.

Uddiyana Bandha

Uddiyana Bandha, also known as the Abdominal Lock, is a yogic practice that supports digestion, tones the abdominal organs, and enhances blood circulation—benefits that are especially valuable during menopause. To perform it, sit cross-legged with your back straight and body relaxed. Take a deep breath in, then exhale completely. After exhaling, gently pull your abdomen inward toward the spine and hold the breath. To release, inhale again and return to your normal breathing pattern. Repeating this practice two to three times can help promote better digestion, improved circulation, and overall well-being.Moola Bandha

Moola Bandha, or the **Root Lock**, is a yogic practice that involves the gentle contraction of the pelvic floor muscles, cultivating inner strength and stability. This technique tones the perineal region and stimulates blood flow to the pelvic area, supporting the health of vaginal and urethral tissues. Regular practice can enhance pelvic health and help prevent issues related to a weakened pelvic floor.

To practice Moola Bandha, sit comfortably in a cross-legged position with your spine upright, hands resting on your thighs or knees. Close your eyes and take a few deep, calming breaths. As you inhale, gently contract the muscles of the pelvic floor—as if trying to stop the flow of urine—engaging the perineal and surrounding muscles. Hold this subtle contraction for a few breaths. As you exhale, slowly release the contraction and return to natural breathing. Repeat this cycle a few times. With consistent practice, Moola Bandha can strengthen the core, support pelvic health, and bring a deeper sense of physical and energetic balance.

Energy Healing

Energy healing- be it through Reiki or chakra balancing, it complements yoga beautifully during menopause. The belief of energy healing is that when the flow of energy in the body becomes obstructed or imbalanced, it can cause physical or emotional disturbances in a person.. Energy healing helps to clear these pathways and brings balance back into the body during the stirring menopausal times because of hormonal changes.

Think of your body as a river: when everything is flowing harmoniously, the water stays crystal clear and smooth. But when it stops moving, stagnation builds up. Similarly, stress, old emotional baggage, or physical discomfort build up are like the stagnant water; they clutter the energy flow. Energy healing cleans up this energetic "debris" so that the energy flows more smoothly; thereby, reducing the symptoms such as anxiety or fatigue.

Another reason yoga and energy healing go so well together during menopause is the building of self-awareness. It's just one of those confusing times when it seems like your body is no longer your own. Yoga calls for a deep connection to your body, helping you tune in rather than feeling out of control. Meanwhile, energy healing reinforces that connection by aligning your energy with your mental and physical states so you feel in tune with yourself. Suddenly, your body isn't foreign anymore!

So, rather than dreading menopause, why not simply embrace this as a time of change? It is yoga and energy healing that could help make this transition not just bearable but a time for self-discovery and renewal. As many a yoga teacher will tell you, this is a time to literally and figuratively "breathe, stretch, and let go" into menopause. Healing and peace are within reach of your fingertips, whether through a soothing yoga session or an energy treatment.

Importance of Energy Healing

Energy healing is what one would consider out of a science fiction novel, but in all actuality, it is an ancient way of keeping one's body and mind balanced. Being somebody open to holistic modes, I ventured into the world of energy healing to help me ease through the severity of the menopause symptoms.

Energy healing relies on the concept that our bodies are composed of energy fields, and when those fields go out of balance, physical and emotional concerns arise. Reiki, acupuncture, and even forms of meditation involve techniques to bring balance back into those fields to facilitate the body's healing and promote wellness.

I'd never heard of energy healing before coming across Reiki, in which a practitioner lays hands directly on or above your body to act as a channel for healing energy. I went in a little sceptical: how was this very passive thing going to make much of a difference? I went into my first session and just felt a really deep level of relaxation, sort of like a weight being taken off my shoulders. It felt like all of the stress and tension in my body could finally be released.

Over time, I did start to feel an improvement in my mood, my sleep, and even hot flashes. Whether it was the power of suggestion, a placebo effect, or whatever, I really am unable to say. But what I do know is that energy healing became a valuable tool in my menopause toolkit.

The other modality of energy healing that helped was acupuncture. This ancient Chinese medicine aims to balance the body by insertion of thin needles into specific points that, according to belief, will restore normal flow or "qi." What worked for me, apparently, was the reduction in anxiety, improved sleep, and mitigated physical discomforts.

Energy healing is probably not for everybody. For me, it offered a way to connect with my body on an altogether deeper level and addressed the disorderly energetic imbalances contributing to my symptoms of menopause.

Just now, I am reminded that our bodies are not only physical; they are also energetic. We can experience true healing when we take care of them in both ways.

Consciousness and Menopause

It's this natural phase in every woman's life, though it can come with many hazards, physical as well as psychological. A consciousness-based approach to menopause focuses not just on the management of symptoms but on deeper healing. The idea is to draw awareness to how our thoughts, emotions, and experiences shape our physical health during this transition.

One of the most common questions is whether or not a daughter will have a similar experience of menopause to the mother. While it is easy to think that the symptoms themselves would follow some form of pattern, at least in the family, the experience as a whole is highly individual. Lifestyle, mental health, and even how we think about our bodies can influence it. With menopause, many women witness changes in their menstrual cycle, aches, and emotional well-being, with fluctuations between varying degrees of intensity and duration. What is crucial here is that all these symptoms are part of an absolutely natural process. Physiologically, the finale of a woman's reproductive cycle has quite objective and tangible premises. So why does it create such turmoil?

Changes with menopause aren't just about the physical state but are very much linked to our emotions and thoughts. It has been proven that our thoughts can change the biochemistry of the body, including how our brain cells, hormones, and nervous systems work. This means the experience of menopause is not only dictated by how we think and feel but also by how we perceive it. Destructive emotions such as shame, anxiety, and stress live not only in our minds; they live in our cells. Guilt and hurtful memories tend to relate to the body on a very deep level. Healing requires purification at all levels: physical, mental, and emotional. Purifying oneself of all those negative influences allows one to receive the deeper healing energies to prepare oneself for entry. This purification process readjusts the body to its original self, and every system tends to work normally.

Women are taught to love and respect their bodies and indeed appreciate them while they are at menopause. This includes an eye for the existence of every organ in their bodies, including female organs. Normally, such systems work to cause shame, especially because of societal pressure. Healing, therefore, comes as a result of conscious love and connection to the body. Meditation can be useful in that regard. Through relaxation techniques, women can internalise their awareness, focus on areas of pain, and send love and light. Ultimately, the experience of menopause can be one of transition, letting go of old emotional baggage and embracing positive appreciation for the body's wonderful functions. Feeding the feminine relationship with her body can make menopause not a time to be uncomfortable but a holistic transition that actually works as one.

With this consciousness-based approach, one is reminded that menopause is not just a natural event but an important point of personal growth emotionally and spiritually. The change in outlook, as well as the development of a loving connection with the body, allows women to transition through this period with most ease and resilience.

Individual Lifestyle Changes and Their Outcomes

As I started making these lifestyle changes- sunlight exposure, grounding, physical activity, and energy healing- I could feel this amazing change within my system. Menopause, which earlier was the toughest challenge for me, was starting to feel manageable. These changes were not about alleviation of symptoms only; they were actually supportive of my body and mind as a whole.

For example, daily sunbathing was not only good for bones but also a habit that was cheerful and energetic.

This form of grounding became a calm ritual to me that made me feel plugged into everything and less stressed. Regular physical activity made me strong and resilient to stress; energetic treatment provided deeper peace and well-being.

These life changes didn't occur in a day, nor was it always easy to stick with them. There were those days when I had missed a workout, forgotten to get outside, or just felt too overwhelmed to practice grounding. But I did learn to be kind to myself, knowing each new day brought along other chances to make healthy choices.

The results? I was empowered, my body was more in tune, and I was better placed to sail through the hard times of menopause. It wasn't about attaining perfection; rather, it was being able to balance, which worked in favour of my health and happiness.

If you are going through menopause, I encourage you to try some of these factors out for yourself. They are easy, accessible, and may really make a big difference in the way you feel. It's not about doing everything perfectly; it's about making small, achievable changes that support your well-being. Most of all, go easy on yourself. Menopause is a process, and with the right life choices, it can be one of growth, self-discovery, and renewed aliveness.

Easy-to-Remember Tips: Chapter 4 – Lifestyle Factors and Menopause

1. **Stay Active** – Incorporate regular exercise into your day.
2. **Quit Smoking** – It impacts your health and accelerates aging.
3. **Limit Alcohol** – Avoid triggers for hot flashes and sleep issues.
4. **Prioritize Sleep** – Create a calming bedtime routine.
5. **Build a Routine** – Balance work, family, and self-care.
6. **Stay Social** – Connect with loved ones to reduce emotional stress.
7. **Practice Gratitude** – Focus on positives to uplift your mindset.

CHAPTER 5

MANAGING MENOPAUSE SYMPTOMS

Menopause is often spoken of as a transition, but if you've experienced it, you know that it can feel more like a fierce rollercoaster. Physical and emotional changes accompanying menopause are more than the natural processes of ageing; they may hit close to home with regard to basic daily living. From hot flashes and night sweats to mood swings and sapping fatigue, these symptoms may be enough in themselves to send you into a dizzy sense of being on a never-stopping Ferris wheel. However, in understanding such symptoms and exploring various modes of treatment, both conventional and alternative, the path through this transition can be eased with more confidence.

This chapter describes the most common menopause symptoms and different treatment options available, and shares some of my personal strategies for dealing with these symptoms. Keep in mind that every woman's menopause is different; therefore, what works for classmate A may not necessarily work for classmate B. The key will be not being too hard on yourself and openness to using different approaches until the best one for you is found.

In-Depth Discussion of Common Menopause Symptoms

First, before looking into the various treatment options and management strategies available for menopausal symptoms, it is necessary to explain what menopause symptoms are, why they present, and how they may vary among different women.

Hot Flashes and Night Sweats

Probably, hot flashes are the best-recognized symptom of menopause. They are described as the sudden sensation of extreme heat that may spread over the face, neck, and chest, often with perspiration and an irregular heartbeat. Night sweats are essentially hot flashes when a person is in bed; this surely could contribute to disrupted sleep from all-night fighting against profuse sweats and then fatigue.

Hot flashes have something to do with your body's thermoregulation system, which is influenced by fluctuating levels of estrogen. The hypothalamus is the part of your brain responsible for controlling your body temperature; it becomes more sensitive to even slight changes in temperature, therefore triggering the hot flash.

Mood Swings and Emotional Changes

Menopause can rightly be termed an emotional roller coaster. You may just feel great one minute, while the next, you are just overwhelmed by feelings of sadness, irritability, or anxiety. Mood changes are influenced by hormonal fluctuation, especially estrogen and progesterone, which affect neurotransmitters such as serotonin and dopamine.

It is quite common during menopause to fall prey to depression or anxiety. These emotions are heightened even more by other life changes that usually accompany this stage, including children leaving home, aging parents requiring even more care, or career changes and alterations in personal relationships. For the body and mind, it is a time of considerable change, and it is quite normal to feel off balance.

Vaginal Dryness and Discomfort

Estrogen decline makes the vaginal tissues much thinner, drier, and less elastic, medically referred to as vaginal atrophy. This condition may cause discomfort, itching, and painful intercourse, among other symptoms. Vaginal dryness, apart from being a nuisance, may provide a fertile ground for urinary tract infections. It is one of those symptoms you may find awkward to share with anyone, yet it is an important thing since it will impact your quality of life.

Sleep Disturbances

Sleep can be very elusive at menopause. Besides night sweats, which usually are the direct culprit, there is more to tell. Increased anxiety, stress, or needing to urinate more frequently can disrupt sleep. And really, insomnia and restless nights just drain you and make you cranky, at an even higher risk for all the other symptoms of menopause. It becomes a self-feeding circle in which bad sleep accentuates everything else.

Gaining Weight and Slowing Down of Metabolism

It's no secret that metabolism usually slows down with age. However, hormonal changes at menopause really accelerate this process and can lead to weight gain. Many women also notice that the extra pounds seem to collect around the midsection, a truly frustrating problem that is also linked to an increased risk of diabetes and heart disease. It is one of the more difficult symptoms of menopause from both a physical and self-esteem standpoint.

Mental Changes

The forgetfulness, lack of focus, and mental fogginess so many women go through at this time is abbreviated as "menopause brain". These changes in cognition are inextricably linked to hormone fluctuations but can also be exacerbated by stress, sleep issues, and general turmoil that comes along with menopause. It is not all in your head: the mental shifts that happen during the menopausal transition are real and quite challenging.

Change in Bone Density

With menopause, the level of estrogen drops tremendously and can make one vulnerable to a rise in all sorts of health changes. One major point of concern is the density of bones because estrogen gives strength to the bones. As the level of estrogen goes down, women are more vulnerable to osteoporosis, which includes thinning of bones, brittleness, and susceptibility to fractures. It is a silent disease, developing without symptoms until a fracture occurs, which is a very serious problem in women in and after menopause.

Change in hair and skin

Lower estrogen levels affect not only bones but also skin and hair. Quite often, hair grows thinner or even becomes more brittle, while some women even start developing facial hair. Skin loses its elasticity and becomes drier, with a tendency to sag and wrinkle. Such changes bother a woman so much because they essentially change her self-image and self-confidence.

Treatment options

There are, therefore, many options of treatments available for menopausal symptoms, both traditional and alternative ones. One of the most common forms of treatment for hot flashes in many hormone therapy programs is called HRT or Hormone Replacement Therapy. It supplements the body with estrogen and progesterone, which reduces symptoms like hot flashes, mood swings, vaginal dryness, and night sweats. HRT is very effective but also carries some risks, which could possibly be associated with heart disease, stroke, and cancer of breast. It is for this reason that a discussion at an in-depth level with your doctor, weighing the benefits and risks, has to be done.

There are non-hormonal alternatives for the uncomfortable ones with hormonal drugs, mainly antidepressants, among them selective serotonin reuptake inhibitors, which can reduce the frequency and intensity of flashes among those women who have associated mood swings. Another useful medication is the antiepileptic agent gabapentin, which also has been shown to ameliorate hot flashes. Antihypertensive drug clonidine may be considered less frequently.

On the other hand, localised kinds are more symptomatic of vaginal estrogen; dryness of the vagina and pain are very much helped by it. This route of medication is able to supply much-needed estrogen to where it is most wanted without as many systemic side effects as oral HRT, inasmuch as administration via creams, pills, or rings directly into the vagina allows for localised action. Medications to help prevent fractures by maintaining or even increasing bone density, such as bisphosphonates or selective estrogen receptor modulators, may be prescribed for at-risk women who have the potential to develop osteoporosis.

Other alternative therapies for menopausal symptoms include herbal supplements, acupuncture, and mind-body therapies. Two of the most commonly used herbal supplements to treat hot flashes are black cohosh and red clover; however, their success does vary among women. Acupuncture, part of traditional Chinese medicine, is the placement of thin needles at specific points on the body. It has also helped some women reduce hot flashes and improve their mood. Yoga, meditation, and breathing exercises are mind-body practices that can help decrease a woman's stress and increase her general well-being at this time in her life.

Bioidentical hormone treatment products that contain hormones identical to those made in the body are sometimes promoted as a more "natural" product than traditional HRT, but their safety and efficacy are not known, and if you choose this option, it is important to be closely guided by a health provider who has experience with bioidentical hormones.

Finding What Works for You

Menopause is different for every woman, and there's simply no one-size-fits-all kind of solution. It's that time, then, when trial and error takes over at the front line to find just the right combination that works for you. Whether your choice of treatment involves conventional medical treatments, alternative therapies, or perhaps some of both, taking care of your health is important during this phase in your life.

You do not have to walk this journey alone. Seek out healthcare professionals, support groups, and loved ones for help and support. You can survive menopause with your head held high if you have the right tools at your fingertips.

Throughout the years, I have tried various approaches to managing my menopausal symptoms. Some are more conventional in treatment; others are more alternative and lifestyle-based.

Here is a glimpse of what worked for me:

Managing Hot Flashes:

Of all symptoms, hot flashes were the most challenging. They seemed to strike at times that were so inconvenient, leaving me flushed, sweaty, and embarrassed. One great way for me to deal with my hot flashes was to wear layered clothing. That way, I could easily remove layers when a hot flash hit.

I also started carrying a small handheld fan in my purse that was an instant cooler. Another thing that helped was the avoidance of triggers: spicy foods, caffeine, and alcohol seemed to decrease the frequency of my hot flashes.

In preparing for bedtime, I invested in moisture-wicking sheets and pyjamas. It made a big difference in being able to sleep comfortably through any night sweats. I also kept a glass of

Had cold water by my bed and practiced deep breathing exercises before sleep to calm my body down.

Mood Swings Easing:

These mood swings were another challenge for me during menopause. Regular exercise, especially yoga, is often used to stabilise my mood. It not only provides physical activity, but in yoga, most of the set comprises deep breathing and meditation, which allows the release of stress and anxiety.

I also made time for self-care consciously. This involved reserving time for activities that I enjoyed, whether it was reading, gardening, or even just taking a long bath. By paying attention to my mental and emotional well-being, I found I could better manage the highs and lows that come with menopause.

Addressing Vaginal Dryness:

The symptom of vaginal dryness was painful and very uncomfortable. I started with a prescription for vaginal estrogen therapy after discussing some options with my doctor, and it made a huge difference. The localised treatment with estrogen helped to restore the moisture and elasticity of the vagina, and the sexual relations felt so much better, and also decreased the risk of urinary tract infections.

Apart from the treatment, I also started using good-quality lubricant; adding an extra layer of comfort during intercourse helped. What was important was that regular application of the lubricant, rather than during sexual activity specifically, kept things moistened.

Improving Sleep:

One of the most frustrating symptoms I had to bear was sleep disturbance. First, to improve my sleep, I instituted a pre-sleep routine to help my body get into a mode for sleep: turn off lights, avoid looking at screens for at least an hour before retiring to bed, and practice deep breathing or progressive muscle relaxation.

I also kept my bedroom as comfortable as possible: cool, dark, and quiet. A good mattress and pillows helped much with making sleep quality better.

Finally, I added melatonin to my regimen, which is a natural sleep aid, to help me fall asleep more easily. Of course, I previously discussed it with my doctor to ensure it was safe for me to take, and it really helps in developing good sleep hygiene.

Weight Gain Management:

Menopausal weight gain can be very frustrating; it is as though no matter what one does, the weight simply refuses to budge. I would find the most helpful strategies for me were a balanced diet complete with whole foods and consistent physical activity.

I started making small, sustainable changes to my diet: a reduction in refined sugars and processed foods, an increase in fruits, vegetables, and lean proteins, and paying attention to portion sizes. I have also made sure to drink enough, as sometimes dehydration masquerades as hunger.

I applied the same no-nonsense approach to exercise: rather than forcing myself into some form of exercise that I hated, I tried looking for what I could enjoy. It is easier this way to repeat the workouts. What worked best was some combination of strength training, maintaining muscle mass and boosting metabolism, and aerobic exercise, which supports the heart and burns calories.

Improving Cognitive Function:

The "menopause brain" was a little less publicised and, quite frankly, incredibly frustrating to deal with. I began adding brain-enhancing foods to my diet, including things like greasy fish with high amounts of omega-3s, leafy greens, and berries.

I also started solving puzzles and playing brain-enhancing games on a routine basis to keep my brain sharp. Minor activities like crosswords, Sudoku, and memory games became enjoyable ways to challenge my brain and hone my focus.

Besides all these tips, being organised and having a daily planner helped me to be in control of my schedule and not be overwhelmed by the stress of forgetting a due date or an appointment.

Taking Care of Bone Health:

Right after being informed about the risk associated with osteoporosis in menopause, I started using some protective measures against the disease affecting my bone health. I started increasing my calcium and vitamin D intake through diet and supplementation. Foods included in my diet were dairy products, leafy greens, and fortified foods.

I also did weight-bearing exercises, like walking, jogging, and strength training, frequently in my routine. Such forms of exercise are able to strengthen bones and maintain bone density.

Finally, I spoke about bone density screening with my doctor and took a bone density test to get an idea about my risk. It gave me peace of mind, taking steps to protect my bones.

Managing the symptoms of menopause is a very personal journey. What works for one woman might not work for another, and that's okay. First and foremost, it means listening to your body, being patient with your actions, and being open to trying new methods.

Whether you are on conventional treatments, alternative therapies, or both, the most important thing is to do what works for you. Never be too scared to seek your healthcare provider, friends, or support groups; importantly, it is not necessary for you to face such a path in life alone.

Menopause is a natural part of life, and while it presents challenges, it can also be a time for personal growth and prioritizing your well-being. By proactively managing your symptoms, you can make positive lifestyle changes that support your overall health.

Easy-to-Remember Tips: Chapter 5 – Managing Menopause Symptoms

1. **Track Symptoms** – Identify patterns to manage them better.
2. **Consider HRT** – Explore hormone therapy with a doctor's advice.
3. **Use Cooling Aids** – Carry a fan or use lightweight clothing for hot flashes.
4. **Focus on Fitness** – Stay active to ease aches and mood swings.
5. **Seek Supplements** – Try vitamin D, magnesium, or herbal remedies.
6. **Stay Patient** – Remember, symptoms can be temporary.

7. **Explore Alternatives** – Consider acupuncture or aromatherapy.
8. **Ask for Help** – Reach out to support groups or counselors if needed.

CHAPTER 6

BONE HEALTH AT MENOPAUSE

As women age, their risk of developing bone-related issues like **osteoporosis** sharply increases, largely because of declining estrogen levels. Maintaining strong bones is crucial for a woman's mobility, independence, and overall quality of life during and after menopause.

This chapter will explore the changes that occur during menopause, focusing on how to prevent osteoporosis. We will also discuss the important roles that diet, exercise, and supplements play in maintaining strong bones. I've included personal experiences to highlight how women can successfully manage their bone health during this transitional phase of life.

The Association Between Menopause and Bone Health

Estrogen levels plunge drastically at the onset of menopause, directly influencing the density of bone. Estrogen essentially maintains the pace of bone resorption with that of bone formation; with estrogen levels declining, bone resorption begins to surpass that of bone formation, and so bone density gradually declines. This can cause osteoporosis, where bones are frail and fragile and likely to break if the condition is not kept under control.

For most women, menopause will trigger the process of bone loss at an accelerated rate. Researchers estimate that the bone density of women may drop as much as 20% within five to seven years after menopause. If left unmanaged, the risk of experiencing osteoporotic fractures of the hips, spine, and wrists becomes exponentially higher. This is, however, not an inevitable fate, and proper management can keep bones healthy into older age.

Vitamin D Levels Change

You need enough **vitamin D** to properly absorb **calcium**, which is essential for strong bones. Unfortunately, as you go through menopause, your body's ability to produce vitamin D from sunlight decreases. This is a problem because lower estrogen levels during this time also reduce the activity of the enzyme that activates vitamin D, which can lead to a significant loss of bone density.

When exposed to sunshine, the body produces Vitamin D, but there are various factors that inhibit this process, including geographical location, skin colour, sunscreen use, and age. These problems, combined with the hormonal changes during menopause, typically cause low vitamin D levels. This, in turn, exacerbates bone loss; thus, monitoring and maintaining optimal Vitamin D levels is critical.

The daily amount for Vitamin D in women over 50 is about 600-800 IU, though the actual needs may be higher. Vitamin D supplements become a prescription during such instances, particularly to women who live in less sunny regions and to those staying indoors more often. It is advisable for all women during menopause to get blood tests regularly to determine if their levels of Vitamin D are sufficient or not.

Osteoarthritis and Menopause

Osteoarthritis is the most common joint disorder that tends to overlap with menopause. Menopausal hormonal changes or a decrease in estrogen might play a significant role in the causation and progression of osteoarthritis. This means that the reduction in estrogen reduces the protective effects on cartilage, making women more susceptible to degenerative joint diseases. Such women may experience increased intensification of the OA symptoms, including enhanced degrees of joint pain, stiffness, and swelling, such as at weight-bearing joints like the knees, hips, and hands. Lifestyle changes in terms of regular exercise and healthy weight maintenance, and sometimes Hormone Replacement Therapy, can help manage OA symptoms during menopause.

Preventing Osteoporosis: Steps to Take

Osteoporosis is a silent disease, which means many years would pass before symptoms occur and a fracture can happen. One can stop it through proactive lifestyle changes, dietary improvements, and regular health check-ups. Here are some key steps women can take to reduce their risk:

- Check on your bone density: DEXA scans monitor bone density at regular intervals that indicate a decline in bone loss early. It is actually a measurement of bone density that provides information on the likelihood of a woman being prone to osteoporosis.
- Adequate Calcium Intake: Most women don't get enough calcium from their diet alone. To help meet your needs, try to include more calcium-rich foods like dairy products, leafy greens, and fortified items such as orange juice and plant-based milk.
- Healthy Vitamin D Levels: Another thing to consider is your Vitamin D level, which your body utilises to absorb calcium. Although sunlight causes your skin to produce more vitamin D, many seafood, including salmon, egg yolks, and even some cereals,

are fortified with vitamin D. Supplements make it much easier for many people to maintain their health levels.

- Exercising: Weight-bearing exercise such as walking, running, and strength training can help you maintain healthy bones. However, resistance workouts that develop muscles also improve bone density, lowering the risk of falls and fractures.
- Avoid smoking and alcohol: Smoking and excessive drinking have been linked to bone loss and fracture risk. Quitting or lowering smoking and drinking is likely to improve bone strength.

Diet's Role in Building Strong Bones

Diet really has a lot to do with keeping our bones healthy, and it only gets increasingly important the older we get. Once menopause strikes, a woman's natural bone density begins to decline, so it's extra necessary to pay attention to everything we eat. A diet high in calcium and other nutrients that are good for the bones will make all the difference in keeping our bones healthy.

First up: calcium-rich foods: Of course, we all know milk, cheese, and yogurt are exceptional sources of calcium. So, what happens if we are lactose intolerant or just don't like the taste of dairy products? No problem! There is a multitude of non-dairy products just as high in calcium. Among these are leafy greens such as kale, spinach, and bok choy; then, there are the calcium-enriched plant-based milks and cereals. It really all comes down to getting enough calcium, from whatever source is most sensible for the person in question.

Tight on the heels is another stalwart defender of bone health: magnesium. Of course, this unsung hero builds bone by acting as a cofactor for enzymes involved in bone formation, stimulating the activity of osteoblasts (bone-building cells), and facilitating the proper absorption and utilization of calcium. And that is not all it does; it also activates Vitamin D, which is another element in the absorption of calcium. Many women do not get enough magnesium; therefore, you will want to know what foods are rich in magnesium. Yeah, that includes almonds, cashews, spinach, and avocados. And they are delicious, and will love your bones right back!

Finally, let's mention Vitamin K. While you are probably familiar with its function in blood clotting, Vitamin K is also an essential nutrient in bone mineralization. It performs the function of regulating the serum calcium level and the delivery of calcium to bones. You can find rich Vitamin K sources in broccoli, brussels sprouts, and green leafy veggies. Adding these to your diet really has a beneficial effect on your bone health.

Building strong bones after menopause isn't just about taking supplements; it's also about eating a healthy diet of naturally supportive foods. By including more greens, nuts, and fortified foods in your meals, you can give your bones the nourishment they need.

One of the key proteins that make up your bones is **collagen**, and its levels naturally decrease as you get older.

Some studies suggest that taking **collagen supplements** can help increase bone density. You can also get collagen from natural sources like bone broth, fish, and poultry. Collagen peptides are another option to support the health of your bones and joints.

Exercise to Strengthen Bones and Aiding Prevention

Exercise is another excellent way to maintain bone health and prevent osteoporosis.

Weight-bearing exercises are particularly effective because they stimulate bone formation. During and after menopause, it's especially important to include activities where your body works against gravity, such as walking, jogging, dancing, or hiking.

Resistant training, either in the form of weight lifting or with resistance bands, is just as important. Exercises that fall into this category actually build muscles, and muscles can be used as an anchor for bones. Another important benefit is balance and coordination, which, when weakened, can lead to an unfortunate fall that does not fracture.

It is advisable that women who have just started doing strength training begin with minimal weights and gradually increase the resistance. For beginners, there are exercises such as squats, lunges, and push-ups, which can be accomplished at home or at a gym and easily modified depending on the level of fitness.

Yoga and Pilates: Also beneficial, in that balance and flexibility reduce the risk of falling. Many women find them not only beneficial to physical health but also useful in dealing with stress and emotional changes associated with menopause.

Supplements Which Support Bone Health

Although diet and exercise form the backbone of maintaining healthy bones, supplements also have a role to play, especially if it becomes impossible to obtain enough from your diet. Some of the most common types of supplements for bone health at menopause include:

This is where supplements come into the strengthening of bones, not just during but also after menopause. Still, like everything else, it's all about finding the balance that best works for one's body.

Calcium is an essential nutrient for bone health, but it's best to get it from your diet if possible. Only take a supplement if your diet is lacking, as getting too much calcium can be harmful and may lead to kidney stones.

The two most common types of calcium supplements are **calcium carbonate** and **calcium citrate**. If you have a sensitive stomach or difficulty with digestion, **calcium citrate** is often the better choice.

Vitamin D is another key player because it helps your body absorb calcium. However, if you live in a place with limited sun or spend a lot of time indoors, you might not get enough. In these cases, most doctors recommend a **Vitamin D3** supplement, as it's the most effective way to increase your blood levels of this important vitamin

Another important mineral is magnesium, available in forms like magnesium citrate, magnesium oxide, and magnesium glycinate. Magnesium is important for maintaining strong bones, but, of course, one would have to consult with a physician about the right amount to take in. Since its overdose can cause digestive problems, getting that dosage right is vital.

Vitamin K2 is the often forgotten companion to calcium and vitamin D. It helps direct calcium to your bones where it belongs, rather than to your arteries, where it can accumulate in dangerous ways. That's probably why you'll find it so often partnered with vitamin D in supplements for bone health: together, they work to increase the density of your bones and clear out the passages of your arteries.

And finally, there is collagen. Though collagen gets a lot of attention for keeping your skin healthy and glowing, this protein also directly plays a role in keeping your bones strong. So, while supplemental forms may be silly-assorted - as powders that can be mixed with morning coffee or your favourite smoothie - many women begin to see improvements in their bone density and ease of motion in the joints after regular use.

In short, supplements can be great additions to your bone health regimen, but approach them with care. It is also best that you consult your healthcare provider so that you're taking the right amount and the right type for your body. Overall, it helps maintain strong and healthy bones up to postmenopausal years.

My Personal Experience

Maintaining bone health in menopause has been a journey for many women, including myself. Of course, I never thought about my bones until I had a minor fall, which ended in my fracture. Well, that was an eye-opening experience.

I started researching ways to make my bones stronger and also prevent further loss of the same. That required that I add some more calcium-based foods to my diet, but surprisingly, I realised exercise played an equal role here. I joined a class with the intention of weightlifting, something I had never thought about before. By surprise, I discovered it to be both empowering and effective. After months of regular strength training, I received better results on bone density tests.

I also began supplementing my routine with Vitamin D and magnesium throughout the winter, as I found out that my blood tests confirmed my levels were within the optimal range. At that stage, I felt pretty confident about continuing those ways of maintaining my health.

In maintaining bone health, the journey for many women is, in essence, finding the right diet, exercise, and supplement balance. For one person, it might work a particular way, but it may not work that way for another. One should, therefore, consult healthcare professionals and try to look at their body's real needs.

In many cases, bone-related issues are an almost silent disease during menopause until one suffers a fracture. In this case, the lowering of estrogen levels, as well as changes that occur with the vitamin D synthesis process, make bones more susceptible to fractures and osteoporosis.

With some focused strategies, such as monitoring of bone density, adequate calcium and Vitamin D intake, exercising, and supplementation, women will have healthy bones even in their old age.

Thus, the setting chapter sharing personal experiences and evidence-based advice calls attention to the proactive approach one needs to have when dealing with bone health. The transition through menopause is possibly not followed by the start of a decline in bone strength, but by being at the very beginning of the path towards it.

Easy-to-Remember Tips: Chapter 6 – Bone Health and Menopause

1. **Boost Calcium** – Include dairy and leafy greens in your diet.
2. **Vitamin D Daily** – Get sunlight or take supplements.
3. **Stay Active** – Do weight-bearing exercises like walking or yoga.
4. **Magnesium Matters** – Eat nuts, seeds, and avocados.
5. **Vitamin K Power** – Add broccoli and spinach to meals.
6. **Limit Smoking and Alcohol** – Protect bone density.
7. **Regular Screenings** – Check for osteoporosis risk.
8. **Collagen Boost** – Consider supplements for joint and bone health.

CHAPTER 7

MENOPAUSE AND SEXUALITY

Menopause is a period of change in a woman's life, accompanied by a variety of physical and emotional symptoms. Sexuality during this stage of a woman's life is one issue that has received a lot of attention lately. Hormones become redistributed and then eventually decreased in many women, bringing about many changes in libido, sexual functioning, and the general sense of intimacy and feelings of connectedness with their partner, which they often report to be confusing but certainly an integral part of the transition through menopause.

While stigma has overshadowed much of the discussion related to menopause and sexuality, openness on the issues is fundamental. It is a fact that life after menopause is not an end to a woman's sexual life but rather an opening for the possibility of renewed connections and intimacies. In this chapter, we shall illustrate changes in libido and sexual function during the menopausal period, common sexual concerns and challenging aspects that may arise, and how women can sustain intimacy in this life stage.

Renewed Sexuality and Sexual Functionality

Menopause triggers a reduction of estrogen, testosterone, and other hormones that regulate sexual function. Such physiological changes, which are regulated by hormone changes, can bring about various physical and emotional changes and thus impact a woman's desire and sexuality. The most common changes include:

- Low Sex Drive: Most women will experience a sudden loss in sex drive once they get close to the menopause stage. This is primarily due to a decrease in testosterone, which is a hormone that regulates sexual desire. Although testosterone is a "male" hormone, women also have the hormone, although in much smaller quantities, and decreases in it often manifest in noticeably weak libido.
- Dryness and Pain in the Vagina: The more estrogen takes a back seat, the thinner, drier, and less elastic the vaginal tissues become. This defines vaginal atrophy, which means sex becomes uncomfortable, painful, or unbearable. In addition, there is no natural lubrication for sex, and sexual activity can only perpetuate irritation. People tend to avoid sexual activities due to fear of pain.

- Changes in Arousal and Orgasm: Some women find it harder to become aroused or to orgasm as they age. Such changes are partly physical, such as reduced blood flow to the genital area, but also psychological, including stress and anxiety that have to do with ageing or body image concerns.
- Psychological and Emotive Changes: Most women undergoing menopause experience mood swings, anxiety, or depression, which could be both psychological and emotional and may impact a woman's sexual sense as well. The emotional burden caused by the symptoms of menopause, involving hot flashes, sleep disorders, and weight gain, contributes to the absence of sexual desire or intimacy.

These changes can be overwhelming, but again, the truth is the body has had a lot of changes through this menopausal transition. Knowing what is happening in the body can leave women working toward finding solutions for these problems and adjusting to this new norm.

Sexual Concerns and Challenges

Such health concerns during menopause, however, play an important role in the general overall well-being of women. Yet women may hesitate and feel even embarrassed to discuss sexual issues with healthcare providers or even their sexual partners. This then leads to many women being isolated with problems that can't be solved. Fortunately, several strategies and treatments are available to counter sexual issues resulting from menopause.

Vaginal Moisturizers and Lubricants

Vaginal dryness is a common menopause symptom that can make intimacy uncomfortable. Fortunately, over-the-counter solutions like **vaginal moisturizers** and **lubricants** can help.

Moisturizers are designed to hydrate the vaginal tissue on a daily basis, providing long-lasting relief and comfort.

Lubricants are designed to reduce friction and make intimate moments more comfortable. When choosing one, look for water- or silicone-based brands. They are less likely to cause irritation and provide extra slipperiness for a more enjoyable experience.

Hormone Replacement Therapy (HRT)

This is another hormone-based medication widely offered to menopausal women who suffer from symptoms such as vaginal dryness, hot flashes, and diminished sexual desire. Supplementing oestrogen with HRT improves sexual performance, makes intercourse more comfortable, and reduces perimenopausal symptoms. There are additional site-specific types of oestrogen therapy, such as creams, rings, or vaginal pills that can be used to treat vaginal atrophy (thinning and inflammation of the vaginal walls). These site-specific treatments limit hormone exposure to the rest of the body, making them a popular alternative for women who wish to relieve vaginal symptoms without disrupting their overall hormone levels.

Hormone Replacement Therapy with Testosterone

Testosterone is not just a male hormone. Many women experience a considerable fall in sex drive as they enter menopause; low levels of **testosterone** might reignite the flames of desire. Nonetheless, contacting a doctor is advised, as testosterone replacement therapy is not suitable for everyone. Once again, the dosage of testosterone supplied must be tailored to minimise potential negative effects while maximising benefits.

Pelvic Floor Exercise

Building your pelvic floor muscles not only helps you control your bladder, but it also improves your sexual experience. For example, Kegel exercises can increase blood circulation to the vaginal region. This will increase sexual enjoyment and lessen pain during intercourse.

And because they are so simple, they are easy to add to your routine; they can be done practically anywhere. Regular pelvic floor exercises can also help avoid urine incontinence, which is a prevalent condition among women after menopause.

Counselling or Therapy

For many women, the psychological and emotional effects of menopause are sexually impactful. Counselling or therapy may be helpful to individuals with anxiety, depression, or marital problems, but a therapist skilled in sexual health or menopause can be particularly advantageous. Couples therapy is also useful when partners seek counselling to cope with issues related to their sexual relationship.

Open Communication with Your Partner

This change in sexual desire or function may be very difficult to discuss, so open communication with your partner is key to a healthy sexual relationship during menopause. Share feelings, concerns, and preferences with your partner so that there can be understanding and support from each other. It may even bring a new way of being intimate and related to one another.

Maintaining Intimacy During Menopause

One of the important sexual health aspects during menopause is intimacy. Intimacy doesn't have to represent sexual intercourse. As the body changes, so can the ways women experience and express closeness with their partners. Emotional connection, touch, and even affection become essential parts of intimacy and can develop relationships at this stage.

Some ways to maintain intimacy through menopause include

- Redefining Intimacy: Changes in sexual function also provide a way of broadening the definition of intimacy that embraces activities that would "increment emotional closeness and bodily affection without anticipation of intercourse." Nonsensual touching like hugging, hand-holding, or giving each other a massage can enhance relationships and intimacy between spouses.
- Making it Comfy: Hot flashes and night sweats make sex seem less enjoyable to some women. By creating a comfortable environment—cooling down the room, using fans, or doing it during a comfortable time of the day—certain discomforts are mitigated, and in any case, intimacy becomes much more enjoyable.

- Quality Time Together: Quality time outside the bedroom can also build an intimacy level. Activities, hobbies, or even just resting together can deepen emotional intimacy. Such emotionally excited couples would naturally get each other sexually.
- Self-Care as Number One: Self-care, physical and emotional, is an important determinant of a healthy sex life. Regular exercise and diet promote sexual function and ability, including libido. Relaxing hobbies such as meditation or yoga help alleviate stress and anxiety and can facilitate the feeling of intimacy.
- Getting Over the Idea: One has to get over the fact that menopause is no state of sexual decay. In fact, several women like being more sexually liberated after menopause when they are free from the taboo fear of pregnancy and societal pressure. Such women might find themselves relishing initiating sex with new freedom.

Personal Reflections about Menopause and Sexuality

Going through menopause, I noticed significant changes in my body. My libido dropped, and vaginal dryness made sex painful. I worried these changes would create distance between my partner and me, fearing it would be the end of the vibrant sex life we once shared.

I also spoke to my doctor, who prescribed low-dose estrogen cream for vaginal dryness. I started to feel better soon after, and sex was comfortable once more. With this and pelvic floor exercises, I could feel I was again in control of my body.

I didn't have to stop having sex during menopause; it just changed. With patience and open communication, I discovered that intimacy can evolve and even flourish in new, unexpected ways at this stage of life

Menopause brings significant changes to a woman's body that can directly affect her sex life and intimacy. While these changes present challenges, they don't have to mean the end of a fulfilling sexual relationship. By addressing issues like **vaginal dryness**, **decreased libido**, and **emotional changes**, women can continue to enjoy intimacy throughout menopause and beyond.

With a mixture of open communication, medical interventions, and an openness to change, women can have many more years of fulfilling sexual pleasures and intimacy well into the postmenopausal years. If menopause signifies the end of intimacy, it opens pathways to reposition and deepen intimacy and pleasure with a partner.

Easy-to-Remember Tips: Chapter 7 – Menopause and Sexuality

1. **Communicate Honestly** – Discuss concerns with your partner.
2. **Use Lubricants** – Reduce discomfort during intimacy.
3. **Hydrate and Moisturize** – Treat vaginal dryness regularly.
4. **Explore Hormone Therapy** – Consult a doctor about HRT.
5. **Practice Kegels** – Strengthen pelvic floor muscles.
6. **Take it Slow** – Rediscover intimacy at your own pace.
7. **Testosterone Therapy** – Seek guidance for low libido.
8. **Educate Yourself** – Understand changes and solutions.

CHAPTER 8

MENOPAUSE AND RELATIONSHIPS

Menopause is a major life transition that affects a woman's body and her relationships. The hormonal shifts that influence physical changes, mood, and overall well-being can also change how a woman interacts with her partner, family, and friends.

However, menopause can also be a time of relationship growth, encouraging couples to communicate more deeply, offer greater support, and adapt to changes as a team.

In this chapter, we shall discuss the impact of menopause on relationships, the role of communication and support in relationships, and personal experiences of changing relationship dynamics during this stage of life.

Effect of Menopause on Relationships

These hormonal changes can bring on a whole range of physical and emotional symptoms, such as hot flashes, irritability, mood swings, fatigue, and even changes in libido. This could make it difficult for couples to be as close and connected as they were when they had the time before, since couples always enter completely new territory.

Some of the ways that this change can affect a relationship are:

- Emotional Stress: Emotional stress tends to be associated with mood swings, irritability, and a sense of sadness or anxiety during the menopausal transition period. This may lead to problems and pressures that begin to mount between a woman and her partner, with overwhelming feelings of disconnection, frustration, and confusion about how partners might help. Misunderstandings or poor communication can bring some sort of tension. Still, if one comes to realise that all these emotional changes are part of the deal during menopause, then such a situation can be handled with much tenderness by both of them.
- Changes in Intimacy: Many women who become less interested in sex or who detest sexual intercourse significantly reduce their level of physical intimacy. Sometimes, this is said to create insecurity or being rejected by one or both spouses as long as the

diminishment in sexual activity is not discussed between partners. However, menopause also gives opportunities for sexual relationships of couples to discover new ways of intimacy, from non-sexual forms of physical closeness to new methods of sexual exploration.

- Rediscovery of Roles: Women almost certainly rediscover their roles in the relationship during this postmenopausal transition. For instance, sometimes, a woman needs to attract much more attention to herself, which then demands a reorganisation of how she and her partners or family manage responsibilities. Maybe one of the reasons why this time can be empowering and challenging is that couples are asked to renegotiate roles concerning how they will support each other at the new milestone in life.

- Rearrangement of Family Relationships: Women's relationships with other family members beyond the romantic partner are also affected. Many changes that occur during the menopausal transition coincide with other major life events, such as offspring moving out of the home or becoming caregivers for elderly members; thus, much of what is happening during this transition will alter the family's dynamics. Perhaps certain individuals will experience an "empty nest" syndrome; feelings of loneliness or loss can place a strain on the way they respond to their partner. Others have caregiving responsibilities, making it even more complicated.

Communication and Support Within Relationships

Communicating with each other and offering support for one another remain important factors in continuing to overcome the challenges of menopause together. This is so only when both parties become willing to communicate openly and find means to support one another, does this transition become a couple's opportunity to strengthen the tie between them.

Important elements in creating communication and support with menopause:

- Open Dialogue: Having an **open dialogue** is key when discussing a sensitive topic like menopause. Both partners should communicate openly about their feelings, expectations, and how the changes are affecting them.
- Women can explain the emotional or physical shifts they are experiencing, while partners can share their own concerns. This helps clear up any

misunderstandings and ensures you both feel you're navigating this journey together.

- Emotional Needs Communication: Because menopause can cause heightened emotions like sadness, anxiety, or anger, it's crucial for women to express their feelings and for their partners to listen without judgment. Understanding that these emotional shifts are part of the process can help partners respond with support instead of frustration.
- Patience and Understanding: There has to be patience and understanding between partners. Menopause can be confusing and frustrating as well. Whatever has to be known has to be reminded that the situation is a passing phase. When they look out for each other, then only can a supportive environment be developed for the relationship to grow stronger in due course.
- Redefining Intimacy: Most couples find that their sex life has changed with the diagnosis of menopause, according to the chapter on menopause and sexuality. Instead of seeing this as a loss, most couples can come to understand that this time affords them an opportunity to redefine intimacy and develop more ways to be intimate with each other. This might include cuddling, holding hands,

and generally doing other things that bring a couple closer together, as opposed to through sexual activity. Openly discussing any distress or sexual matters can also lift the burden and prevent feelings of rejection.

- Professional Counseling: In some instances, the hurdles that are brought by menopause may be so massive that they cannot be dealt with on their own. Professional counselling by a therapist or counsellor may be of many benefits in coming to terms with issues of life during and after menopause. This way, couples will be able to sit down and deliberate about their fears and may even be able to work better through emotional pitfalls and devise strategies for a healthy relationship during menopause.

While menopause can present challenges in a relationship, it also offers a unique opportunity for couples to grow closer. The physical changes can be difficult at first, but with open communication and mutual support, you can navigate this transition together. By embracing these changes and finding new ways to maintain intimacy and closeness, many couples emerge from menopause with a stronger, deeper bond than ever before. It all comes down to patience, understanding, and a willingness to adapt as a team.

Easy-to-Remember Tips: Chapter 8 – Menopause and Relationships

1. Acknowledge Emotions – Accept mood swings.
2. Talk Openly – Share feelings.
3. Show Empathy – Support, not frustration.
4. Redefine Intimacy – Explore closeness.
5. Adjust Roles – Balance responsibilities.
6. Seek Help – Use therapy if needed.
7. Self-Care – Prioritize your well-being.

CHAPTER 9

MENOPAUSE AND CAREER

Menopause is a natural point in a woman's life, but more often than not, it often falls at a time in her career when she is reaching a crucial point. Women now, as they reach menopause or transition into postmenopause, are precisely at their best in terms of careers, with substantial leadership responsibilities, peak career growth, or transitions. Still, women who have even slight menopause symptoms, which may be anything from hot flashes and lack of energy to emotional changes such as mood swings or anxiety, face much more complicated circumstances at work and in life. But with the right strategies, women can work and even further their professional careers.

In this chapter, we will explore the balance between work and menopause, strategies for managing work-related challenges, and personal experiences that reflect the variety of paths women take during this phase of life.

Balancing Work and Menopause

Managing the symptoms of menopause and a successful career at the same time can be challenging.. Large populations of women are caught in the middle of needing to balance their individual health needs with the demands of being in a very high-stress work environment. While some work environments have become increasingly more understanding of women's health issues, there's still much stigma and a lack of understanding of issues related to menopause.

This would coincidentally be the peak point of their careers for most women. They would either be in leadership roles, managing teams, or handling responsibilities. The added challenge of fluctuating hormones, mood swings, and fatigue creates tension. Symptoms such as brain fog or reduced concentration may affect productivity, leading to anxiety about job performance.

These challenges are real, but women have learned through time and through stressful situations how to balance work life and menopause, change their routines, and develop coping mechanisms. It's that creativity that creates a balance between professional and healthful living.

Coping with Work-Related Issues

There are many strategies available to manage the overlap between menopause and work, and women can achieve both performance and well-being through such flexible approaches.

- Communication in the Workplace: Although the stigma of menopause is still there, openness and being honest with supervisors or peers about this situation may lead to support. When productivity slows down because of symptoms, adjusting work or communicating with colleagues at the workplace can become a determining factor for change. Some companies recently took up menopause-friendly policies as they realized that work-life balance benefits the person who is going through the transition as much as it benefits the organisation.
- Self-Care and Mindfulness: One simple way to integrate self-practices into daily life during menopause is through self-care. Yoga, meditation, and deep breathing exercises are excellent tools for mood regulation and dealing with stressors. This can be especially useful for someone in a high-stress job. Many women find that stepping outside for some mindfulness or stretching during the day keeps them centered.

- Flexible Work Schedules: There needs to be flexibility. Women who have very severe symptoms benefit by having a flexible work schedule or being allowed to work from home. This would provide the means to care for other symptoms of fatigue and insomnia without the burden of a 9-to-5. For those in more leadership positions, task delegation or accommodation of work hours can help these women retain their role of leadership.
- Nutrition and Hydration: I have also talked to you about the role food and nutrition play in Chapter 3.
- Physical Activity: As we discussed earlier, exercise reduces stress, helps sleep, lessens the impact of hot flashes, and, in addition to miserable feelings, reduces joint discomfort from tender joints and muscles.
- Cognitive Behavioral Therapy (CBT): For many of us women, it is common to experience anxiety, irritation, or emotional upset during menopause. Going to a professional for CBT can be a great help for you during this time. Cognitive behavioural therapy is a type of psychotherapy that helps people find and break negative thoughts and patterns.
- Access to support networks: Working life can dramatically change when women go through

menopause. Therefore, having support networks in the workplace really makes a difference for people going through this transition. Women may benefit by just confiding in coworkers or forming small groups where they may share experiences. In some cases, just knowing that you are not alone in dealing with the challenges of menopause can be a relief. Women should also seek support outside of work through online forums or local support groups.

Menopause is a natural process that occurs in every woman's life. However, not every woman faces the same problems. The first step to understanding that you are suffering through menopausal symptoms is to accept and watch out for the signs of changes in yourself.

My daily routine

A balanced daily routine can help a woman cope with the symptoms of menopause and lead a healthy life. In most cases, mindful practices are part of the routine, such as maintaining a healthy diet, exercise, and activities that reduce stress. These habits provide a friendly structure that makes the change easy for someone as they go through the middle period of a woman's life, thereby making them live a quality life.

Time	Activity
5.30 am	Wake up Do bed exercises, such as Dry brushing for lymphatic drainage Neck exercises Silent meditation for 5 minutes Oil Pulling
6.00 am	Exposure to rising sun along with grounding exercise/walking
6.15 am	Practicing inner engineering by Sadhguru (Isha Foundation, Coimbatore) for 45 mins
7 am	I take a glass of water after putting my positive intentions into it.
7.15 am	I have my bulletproof coffee.
7.30 am	Hot and cold showers
8. 30 am	Prepare my to-do list for the day

Time	Activity
9.30 am	Have my breakfast (as discussed in the previous chapter)
10.30 am	Ready, set, get started with my work
1.00 pm	Lunch

3.00 pm	I do my exercises
4.00	Resume work
5.30 pm	Go for a walk in the nearest park
6.00 pm	Early light dinner, followed by some 'me' time
9.30 pm	Retire to bed

Therefore, in conclusion, all career women experiencing menopausal symptoms should come up with an action plan for a support system, both at the workplace and in the family. Open communication with colleagues and family members, setting boundaries, and perhaps establishing a constant daily routine can lead to meaningful differences during this stage of their lives. To summarise, the most important thing for working women going through menopause is to establish a solid support network at work and at home. Open communication with coworkers, family, and friends can promote understanding and establish an environment of empathy and cooperation. Equally crucial is developing a consistent regimen that includes self-care, diet, exercise, and stress management that is suited to your specific requirements during this time. Women can face this transformative era with confidence by striking a balance between professional commitments and personal well-being, allowing them to maintain productivity and a sense of fulfilment in both their careers and personal lives.

Easy-to-Remember Tips: Chapter 9 – Menopause and Career

1. **Plan Ahead** – Prepare for energy dips during work hours.
2. **Communicate at Work** – Share challenges with trusted colleagues.
3. **Use Flexibility** – Adapt your schedule if possible.
4. **Stay Organized** – Use planners to manage brain fog.
5. **Take Breaks** – Incorporate short rests to recharge.
6. **Create a Support Network** – Seek mentorship or peer groups.
7. **Embrace Wellness** – Practice mindfulness or meditation.
8. **Advocate for Yourself** – Speak up about needs or adjustments.

CHAPTER 10

LOOKING AHEAD: POST-MENOPAUSE

Something I discovered during my study is that the age at which menopause starts varies significantly for different women, and there are no discernible patterns of any form related to age. Most women experience menopause somewhere in the range of 50 to 55 years of age. That is the most typical range. It happens because the body naturally experiences declining reproductive hormones, especially estrogen, and the menstrual cycles eventually cease altogether.

On the other hand, a significant percentage of women-37.5% -- approach menopause a little early, and this happens when they are between 45 and 49 years old. The cause for early menopause could be genetic predisposition, smoking, some type of medical treatment, or even one's overall condition. The women would then begin experiencing symptoms of menopause in their mid-to-late 40s, like hot flashes, mood swings, and changes in the menstrual cycle.

Finally, around 12.5 per cent of women experience menopause at age 55 and beyond. Late menopause may be associated with several characteristics, such as increased body weight, genetics, or prolonged exposure to estrogen, such as in the case of heavy bleeding. Some may think of this as an advantage in terms of fertility, but it carries another risk of late menopause in the form of a higher risk for breast or ovarian cancer.

The wide variation in the timing of menopause underscores how unique this transition is for every woman, shaped by her individual health, lifestyle, and genetic background.

This means postmenopause is the final stage of the menopause process. Post-menopause is said to be when a woman has not had her menstrual period for twelve consecutive months. Menopause is said to begin with this stoppage, but post-menopause is that period beyond this stage, and it has often brought with it a newfound freedom and, in certain ways, a change.

This chapter will explore what life is like after menopause: what are the physical and emotional changes, new opportunities and challenges, and how to excel during this time. For most women, post-menopause is a liberating time of self-discovery and increased appreciation for what is important: health and well-being.

Life After Menopause: New Beginning

Many women feel uncertain about life after menopause. On one hand, it can bring relief from frustrating symptoms like hot flashes, night sweats, and mood swings. On the other hand, it marks a new phase where changing hormone levels can affect the body in different ways

For many women, however, the post-menopause years feel like a renewal. After the hormonal fluctuations subside, their bodies stabilize. Women often report having more energy, better mental clarity, and a new sense of freedom from the ups and downs of their menstrual cycle. It's a time to focus on health, relationships, and personal passions with a clear vision of who they are and what they want.

Physical Changes in Post-Menopause

Though the major hormonal changes are finally stable, postmenopause brings physical alterations into play. Understanding these and actively working on their management is key to being healthy and fulfilling in life after menopause.

- Bone Health: Estrogen holds an extremely significant role in maintaining the strength of bones. Removal of this hormone at the time of menopause may well increase the risk of osteoporosis. It is thus recommended that women in post-menopause take such precautions towards their bone health. These include rich calcium diets and vitamin D supplements, bone-strengthening exercises, and even hormone replacement therapy or drugs prescribed by healthcare providers in a few instances.
- Heart Health: The decline of this protective estrogen leaves the post-menopause woman at greater risk for cardiovascular disease. Lifestyle habits like regular exercise, a balanced diet, and stress management will greatly reduce those risks. Cholesterol levels and blood pressure should be checked regularly, and a healthcare professional should be consulted to discuss preventive measures.
- Skin and Hair: Estrogen deficiency results in loss of skin elasticity and moisture; it tends to become dry and wrinkle-persistent, and hair is thinning. Most women attend to their skin by hydrating enough, protecting themselves from the sun, using moisturising products, and maintaining a healthy diet consisting of antioxidants that contribute to healthy hair and skin.

- Weight Management: Most of the women experience weight gain after menopause. In particular, they tend to gain weight in their abdominal area. However, it can be controlled simply by eating a healthy diet combined with exercise. Of course, exercise can help in weight management. It also raises energy, improves mood, and increases overall well-being.
- Sexual Health: Libido will fluctuate, and vaginal dryness can be severely uncomfortable; however, some women discover themselves sexually liberated from the requirement for contraception. Many will have reduced libido after menopause, and others discover they are now sexually liberated without fear of pregnancy. Moisturisers, lubricants, and often hormone therapy can reduce pain during sexual intercourse.

Emotional Changes: A Change in Point of View

Just as the body changes with age, so do the mental bodies. During their post-menopausal years, women often turn inward in quest of self-evaluation and reassessment of priorities. For many, this phase is characterised by emotional readiness and authority. Now freed from the hormonal turmoil of menopause, women are often able to be more truly in command of their emotions and psychology.

- Emotional Balance: The mood swings and anxiety that can often accompany perimenopause have diminished in post-menopause, leaving a calmer and more emotionally stable woman. Women often report becoming more centered and at peace with themselves during this stage.
- Rediscover Life Purpose: For many people, the post-menopausal transition is a good time to reassess life goals or passions again. Children are grown and either well established in their professional lives, moving into new ones, or free from stereotypical reproductive roles; often, women rediscover passion or projects or even change careers at such an age. Post-menopause gives an opportunity for individual transformation. Whether travelling, starting a new business, volunteering, or pursuing an artistic passion, many women regard this phase of life as their time to focus on themselves and the things they have always wanted to do. People are freed from responsibility in child-rearing and even from high-stakes careers. Such individuals can continue to explore whatever opportunities are in life.

- Self-Esteem: For some, the post-menopausal years boost self-esteem. The pressure to conform to societal standards of youthfulness decreases, and women can take pride in their age. Most achieve a profound sense of self-acceptance and self-esteem that they may never have felt before in life.

Opportunities and Challenges in Post-Menopause

While post-menopause brings a lot of possibilities and personal growth, it cannot be without its challenges. Women need to learn to live this new stage of life very optimistically but with down to earth strategies for their health and emotional well-being.

Relationships at the New Living Conditions: Life exists after menopause. It includes relationships, which are a part of that new life. Sometimes, this new relationship brings women closer to their spouses as they have more time to continue investing in their relationship.

Financial Planning and Security: This can be a time when financial objectives need to be revisited following menopause. With retirement around the corner, women should ensure that they have something in place for themselves in the future. That may include managing and advising investments and savings, and may even consider long-term care plans. For one, it may mean working right up to retirement or finding new income sources, while for others, it may mean enjoying the fruits of a just-ended career and planning for a quiet post-retirement period.

Coping with Family Transition: Most post-menopausal women are affected by transition in family life because the children leave to live elsewhere, grow to be independent, and gradually initiate their families of their own. This is often a time full of joy in being a grandparent, yet it is also a time marked by potential grief and voids as the previously noisy nest becomes quieter. Finding ways to stay connected with others and discovering a new sense of purpose in family relationships can help ease this transition for them.

Embracing the Next Chapter

This is the beginning of a new life after menopause. Since the hormonal rollercoaster has stopped, women can begin to live for health, hobbies, relationships, and self-improvement. Although, of course, post-menopause isn't always an easy time either, it offers tremendous potential for renewal and empowerment. Women can navigate through this phase with confidence, looking at the opportunities given but taking proactive measures so that they stay in both physical and mental health.

Post-menopause is not an end; it is a fresh new beginning in life.

Easy-to-Remember Tips: Chapter 10 – Looking Ahead: Post-Menopause

1. **Stay Active** – Keep moving to maintain physical health.
2. **Eat Well** – Focus on nutrient-rich, balanced meals.
3. **Celebrate Freedom** – Embrace the end of menstrual cycles.
4. **Maintain Relationships** – Keep fostering meaningful connections.
5. **Stay Curious** – Explore hobbies or passions.
6. **Prioritize Self-Care** – Make your health a top priority.
7. **Be Vigilant** – Continue regular health check-ups.
8. **Keep Learning** – Educate yourself about post-menopause wellness.